THE Secret TO Skinny

How Salt Makes You Fat
and the 4-Week Plan to
DROP A SIZE AND GET HEALTHIER
with Simple Low-Sodium Swaps

Tammy Lakatos Shames, R.D.
Lyssie Lakatos, R.D.
The Nutrition Twins

Health Communications, Inc.
Deerfield Beach, Florida

www.hcibooks.com

Disclaimer: The information contained in this book is not intended as a substitute for the advice and/or medical care of a physician. It is recommended that you consult with your physician before embarking on any eating, exercise, or lifestyle regimen.

Library of Congress Cataloging-in-Publication Data

Lakatos, Lyssie.
   The secret to skinny : how salt makes you fat, and the 4-week plan to drop a size and get healthier with simple low-sodium swaps / Lyssie Lakatos and Tammy Lakatos Shames.
      p. cm.
   Includes bibliographical references and index.
   ISBN-13: 978-0-7573-1351-6
   ISBN-10: 0-7573-1351-5
   1. Salt-free diet.   2. Weight loss.   I. Shames, Tammy Lakatos.   II. Title.
RM237.8.L35 2009
613.2'85—dc22

                                                                        2009025601

HCI, its logos, and marks are trademarks of Health Communications, Inc.

Publisher: Health Communications, Inc.
            3201 S.W. 15th Street
            Deerfield Beach, FL 33442–8190

Cover design by Larissa Hise Henoch
Interior design and formatting by Lawna Patterson Oldfield

To Summer and Riley

Contents

Acknowledgments

Special thanks to our wonderful editor, Allison Janse, whose incredible vision and tireless efforts helped to mold this book. We feel so lucky to have had the opportunity to work with you, and we truly couldn't ask for a more insightful and dedicated editor. Thank you. Thank you to our amazing literary agent, Laura Dail, of Laura Dail Literary Agency, for always believing in us and for working your magic to make this all happen.

Our warmest thanks to everyone at HCI, especially to Carol Rosenberg and Candace Johnson for guiding this book through to its finish; to Kim Weiss for your fabulous PR expertise; and to Tonya Woodworth for your fantastic eye for detail.

To the amazing Jessica Fishman Levinson, M.S., R.D., C.D.N., thanks for your amazing support, your hard work, and your nutrition expertise. Without your fantastic writing contributions, this book would not be what it is.

To Theresa Quadrozzi, thanks for your inspiration, encouragement, and writing expertise.

Thank you to all our clients who have taught us how to take nutrition science and turn it into practical, everyday advice, even for those with the most hectic of schedules.

To all of the great chefs who contributed their delicious recipes to our book, we are so grateful.

To Lou D'Amico, a huge thanks for keeping us creative and for always helping us to find a "salternative."

Another big thank you to Sara Joseph for your support and for being so on top of your PR game—and, of course, thank you for being such a great friend.

On a personal note, thanks to our incredible friends and family for always being there for us. Without all of you, this journey would not be the happy experience that it is.

Thanks to Mom and Dad for your love and support in everything that we do—without you both, we would never be where we are today.

And to Tammy's husband, Scott, thank you for your constant support and for helping Tammy to get through the long hours.

Last, but certainly not least, thanks to Tammy's twin daughters, Summer and Riley, for always making us smile, always helping us to keep things in perspective, and reminding us what we value most. You both truly are an inspiration.

Introduction

As registered dietitians and certified personal trainers, we've spent more than a decade helping thousands of clients get healthy and achieve the bodies they longed for. Not only do our clients typically reach their dream weights, more important, they *keep* the pounds off. Our clients have kissed yo-yoing dieting good-bye and have embraced their new slender bodies for life.

While our core weight-loss beliefs haven't been swayed by fads, we continually refine our methods to find innovative ways to help our clients attain maximum results. Our most recent diet discovery compelled us to write this book because we found what we consider the missing link when it comes to weight loss. Many new clients came to us frustrated from months or years of dieting without substantial or lasting results, convinced that they couldn't lose the stubborn pounds because of too many carbs, too little cardio, or not enough stomach crunches. And although at times they were right, after analyzing their habits, we came to realize that more often than not, something else was flying under the radar, hindering them from achieving the body they wanted.

The culprit? It's seemingly innocent, and often invisible, so most people don't pay it any attention when it comes to weight loss. But if you're trying to lose weight, it's one of the nastiest four-letter words:

S-A-L-T. And, as we will explain, our experience proves that if you learn to drop the salt, you will drop a size—or more—and add years to your life.

Salt is ubiquitous: Most of us unknowingly consuming 75 percent of our sodium intake from prepared foods, not from the saltshaker. According to a 2008 *Time* magazine article, typical American adults eat 50 percent more salt than we did in the 1960s—*more than twice the amount that our bodies can process.* Manufacturers sneak salt into everything, especially the "healthy" foods that we dutifully eat while trying to be "good"—everything from low-fat salad dressings and packaged diet entrees, to lean meats and soups, and wheat breads and cereals that are touted as healthy.

Why Excess Salt = Excess Weight

Once inside your body, salt wreaks havoc on your waistline. In fact, a 2007 study published in *Obesity Research* shows that high-salt diets are directly associated with more fat cells in the body. Even worse, salt makes the fat cells you already have become denser. Thicker fat cells? *No, thank you!*

If you eat a lot of salt, your kidneys have to work overtime to excrete the excess. In the Western world, "excess" is an understatement. Most people get 4,000 to 6,000 milligrams of salt *per day,* far exceeding the 1,500 to 2,400 milligrams that the body can handle. No matter how hard your kidneys work to reduce body sodium, salt builds up in the tissues, causing salt-saturated cells and salt toxicity. Excess salt damages cells. And damaged cells don't function at their best. This means all bodily processes will suffer, including your metabolism and your ability to burn fat and repair muscle. A high-salt diet hardens your arteries, making it more difficult for fat-burning oxygen to get to your cells. Less oxygen to your cells means a less efficient metabolism, and therefore less fat burned overall.

In addition, salt *increases* food cravings. Obviously, hunger is the last thing you want when trying to trim down. This may be one reason research shows that diets high in salt lead to obesity.

Salt and the Dreaded Bloat

If you ingest more salt than you need, you'll never beat the bloat because a high-salt diet makes you retain water. Even when you lose a significant amount of weight and lose the body fat you hoped to, you will often still feel puffy and bloated. Why? Sodium attracts and holds water, which increases your blood volume. Increased blood volume means your body expands, making you bigger and thicker. If you eat a lot of salt, you can be holding as much as 5 to 10 pounds of extra water. That's the equivalent of ten to twenty 8-ounce bottles of water! Even if you are lean, this extra water will make you look and feel puffy and distended. This is probably not the look you are going for. If this isn't enough to make you want to slash the salt, consider how salt is putting your health at risk.

Salt and Your Health

For years, people believed that salt could only cause disease if it was raising blood pressure. The thinking was that as long as your blood pressure remained in the normal range, no harm was done. The truth is that chronically overconsuming salt damages your heart, brain, kidneys, and arteries. High blood pressure is a very common *symptom* of that damage. However, the absence of one symptom (such as high blood pressure) does not mean that the disease process isn't present. Even if your blood pressure is not high, you may still have the underlying disease—salt toxicity. Many of us with normal blood pressure have a false sense of security. But the reality is that the more salt we consume, the greater the strain on the heart. The heart is the most important muscle. If it's not functioning properly, blood and nutrients can't get to the muscles, tissues, and organs efficiently. Over time, salt's strain on the heart damages the entire body, even without a diagnosis of hypertension. Most people realize that high blood pressure is a major risk factor for heart disease. High cholesterol and hardened arteries are also risk factors. But did you know that if you lower your salt intake throughout your life, high cholesterol and hardened arteries pose less of a threat? Salt directly contributes to cardiovascular disease, the leading cause of death in the United States, sending more Americans to an early grave each year than all cancers combined. And this is just the beginning. In fact, salt poses such a threat that worldwide action is finally being taken. Salt is rising to the top of the world's health agenda; every major health agency, including the World Health Organization and the National Academy of Sciences, has recommended drastic reductions in sodium consumption.

Eat less salt and you lower your risk of stomach cancer, osteoporosis, and kidney stones. Plus, you'll be keeping the rest of your body in better working order. So if you want to gain control of your weight and your health, you need to become salt-savvy. We've helped our clients slash the salt, and we can help you, too. It's your turn to attain the trim and healthy body of your dreams. We're going to help you to lose the salt—and the weight—for good.

The Secret to Skinny

The Secret to Skinny provides you with a detailed road map to get you in top shape. Not only will you look tight and toned, you'll kick the bloated feeling for good. You'll start by measuring your weight, waistline, butt, hips, and thigh size, and you'll have your blood pressure and cholesterol level measured (see Appendix IV for a chart to track your progress). Ask your doctor to take your blood pressure and measure cholesterol. Finding your cholesterol requires a simple blood test. After four weeks on our plan, you'll remeasure. You'll lose at least 10 pounds (likely more, if you have a lot of weight to lose), drop at least one clothing size (likely more), and lose at least an inch in your waist, hips, and thighs. You're also likely to see a significant improvement in your blood pressure and cholesterol level. For every three points you lower your blood pressure, you'll lower your risk of dying from a stroke by 8 percent and lessen your chance of dying from heart disease by 5 percent.

Your Weight-Loss Weapons: Slimmers, Flushers, and Anti-Bloaters

You'll build your meals and snacks with key foods that we've categorized as "Green Light" foods: Slimmers, Flushers, and Anti-Bloaters. These foods are your best friends when it comes to weight loss. Why? Slimmers provide your body with energy, and they're packed with important vitamins that help turn food into usable energy. High in fiber and nutrients, or full of lean protein, Slimmers provide long-lasting energy without the sugar highs or crashes that make you prone to bingeing. Flushers and Anti-Bloaters are high in water content and fiber. They prevent constipation (and the bloat that goes with it!); they help excrete excess salt from your body; and they keep you feeling full longer.

In addition to the Green Light foods, we'll also open your eyes to the biggest weight-loss saboteurs that might be lurking in some of the foods you eat every day. We'll reveal the "Red Light" Pluggers, Bloaters, Chubbers, and Flabbers—foods which cause weight gain, bloating, and less than stellar health over time.

You'll begin with the Jumpstart Plan, a ten-day, hard-core, quick-results plan. This plan is not recommended for long-term use because you would need a lot of willpower to stick with it. However, this Jumpstart phase is great when you want to look your leanest for an upcoming event, and it's a great fallback plan if you feel yourself slipping and gaining weight (after the holidays, for example). Once you complete this phase, you will move on to phase 2, the Maintenance Plan, which allows more food choices, daily indulgences, and a higher calorie intake. For both plans, we provide daily menus and delicious recipes.

We will also give you salt-slashing and calorie-saving tips and show you how many pounds these changes will save you over the course of a year. These simple "salternatives" can also add years to your life. For example:

- Ditch your daily afternoon bottle of Snapple ice tea (which happens to have 200 calories and 20 milligrams of sodium) and opt for green tea (which has zero calories and is sodium free). You'll save about 20 pounds a year and eliminate 16 days' worth of sodium!
- Twice a week, whether at home or at a restaurant, choose rice (even white rice) instead of rice pilaf and save 4.5 pounds per year and eliminate 36 days of sodium!

Finally, we'll show you how to make your food taste delicious without adding belt-bursting salts or fats, and we'll provide you with a repertoire of low-sodium recipes to incorporate into your healthier, happier, and slimmer life.

How to Use This Book

Consider this your guide to getting and staying lean. Below you'll find brief chapter descriptions so you can dive into the parts of the book that you feel will benefit you the most.

In chapter 1 you'll learn why salt is making you fat and creating disease; hopefully you'll be fired up to begin the Jumpstart Plan, which will get you the quick results you want. In chapter 2, we introduce you to the Green Light foods that will blast the fat and bloat and keep it off, and we teach you how to build your meals and snacks on the Jumpstart Phase. If you don't care for meal-planning, you can simply follow the ten days of Jumpstart Menus that we provide in chapter 3 on page 47.

Chapters 4 and 5 will give you real-world hints, tips, and tricks to successfully navigate a sodium-laden world at home, at the supermarket, and while you're out and about. Chapter 6 details the Maintenance Plan, which allows you more flexibility with food while still ensuring a consistent, healthy weight loss. You'll learn the additional foods you can incorporate into your diet, including Yellow Light foods, which aren't as healthy as the Green Light foods, and you'll find two weeks of Maintenance menus in chapter 7. While on the Maintenance Plan—which you'll hopefully adopt for life—you'll get to indulge in two daily servings of Red Light foods, which are decadent but can be detrimental to your weight loss goals if you overindulge; we detail these Pluggers, Bloaters, Chubbers, and Flabbers in chapter 8.

For optimal results, we recommend getting active, and in chapter 9 we provide guidance to help you make your body toned and tight. For your convenience, you'll find our favorite low-sodium recipes in chapter 9 and lists of popular brand-name Green Light, Yellow Light, and Red Light foods in the Appendixes.

Now, let's get to the Secret to Skinny. . . .

Chapter 1

What's Salt Got to Do with Your Weight and Health? More Than You Think

All set to go with *The Secret to Skinny* plan? Before we explain how dropping the salt can help you drop a size, you might want to better understand what too much salt does to your health and your appearance and therefore why it's so important to stick to the plan.

Many people are well aware of the health problems that too much salt can cause, including high blood pressure and cardiovascular disease. But most people aren't aware of how excess salt contributes to weight gain.

Sodium, along with other minerals such as calcium, magnesium, chloride, and potassium, is an electrolyte that helps keep your metabolism running, ensures proper flow of nutrients and waste into and out of your

> **6 Reasons to Drop the Salt**
> - Salt increases the number of fat cells in your body
> - It makes the fat cells you have fatter
> - Salt prevents your metabolism from burning fat as it should
> - It increases insulin resistance
> - It makes you hungrier and thirstier
> - Salt makes it more difficult for fat-burning oxygen to blast the fat in your fat stores

body, and maintains the acid-base (pH) balance in your blood. If you get too much sodium, you create electrolyte imbalances that throw your body off-kilter. This means your metabolism can't function at its peak, and you can't burn as much fat as you should.

Excess salt also negatively affects insulin, a hormone that helps transport sugar out of the blood and into the muscles and tissues for energy. This means that insulin can't do its job, so sugar builds up in the blood, damaging vessels and making it difficult for fat-burning oxygen to flow to cells and melt fat. Making matters worse, when people gain weight, especially in the abdominal area, they can become insulin resistant. This means their bodies don't respond well to insulin. In response, the pancreas secretes more insulin, which in time can result in diabetes. With higher insulin levels, not only does your body store more fat, but your kidneys will have a harder time getting rid of salt, which can lead to electrolyte imbalances, high blood pressure, and bloating.

Have you ever found it hard to stop eating after a handful of salty chips or salted nuts? Your willpower wasn't an issue. The fact is salty foods increase your thirst and hunger, making it more likely that you'll consume calories you don't need. And, as we mentioned in the Introduction, recent research shows that a high-salt diet causes fat cells to become denser, which is not going to help you win the battle of the bulge.

Bloating and Appearance

In addition to weight gain, too much sodium can take a toll on your appearance, including causing a puffy, tired-looking face. Ever notice that after a meal filled with salty foods (think soy sauce, smoked fish or meat, French fries, or chips) your stomach is distended and you weigh more the next morning? That's your body's reaction to eating too much salt. The retention of extra water and fluid leads to major bloating. Even if you're skinny, you'll still look bloated and puffy from all the excess fluid.

Think you can hide the bloat with your clothes? You may be able to if you're a fashion genius, but you can't hide it on your face. Think about how people look when they have a hangover after too much alcohol. They wake up feeling tired and headachy, and

> **Salt** is **not** the same thing as sodium. Salt contains sodium and chloride. However, to simplify, we use the terms "salt" and "sodium" interchangeably since most people need to reduce sodium, and the best way to do it is to cut back on salt.

when they look in the mirror, the result is on their face. It's the same with a "salt hangover." (See our Emergency Salt Hangover Remedies in chapter 4 on page 78.)

Excess salt damages your cells, which means you won't look as good as you usually do because injured cells on the inside lead to damage on the outside. What's more, most salty, processed foods lack essential nutrients (B vitamins and zinc) that help your body maintain optimal health, and they also lack the antioxidants (vitamins A, C, and E) that help fight off damaging free radicals. Too many salty, processed foods increase inflammation in your body, which can then lead to red and irritated skin and puffy bags under the eyes, as well as serious degenerative diseases.

Heart Disease

Salt-filled foods can lead to cardiovascular disease, not only from high blood pressure, but also from increased fat and cholesterol intake. Most of the salt Americans get comes from processed food, which is full of fat, cholesterol, and calories. Not only do these fats attach to your waist, hips, and thighs, they also clog and harden your arteries and make it more difficult for oxygen to get to your cells. When oxygen can't get to your cells, not only can't you burn fat, but you are also at higher risk for a heart attack. When your heart pumps blood through the blood vessels, oxygen and nutrients are delivered to your cells, and waste products are removed (you get an energized body, glowing skin, nourished muscles, and increased fat burning). As it circulates, your blood exerts a force against the walls of the blood vessels, and this force is known as your blood pressure (BP). Problems occur when your blood vessels get clogged up. This can happen from eating large amounts of fat and cholesterol, but too much salt intake is also a major culprit in clogging the pipes. Since excess salt intake leads to excess water in the blood, there is more pressure in your blood vessels, and your heart has to work harder. This is what we call *high blood pressure* or *hypertension*.

If your blood pressure is between 120/80 and 139/89, you have prehypertension, which means you're likely to develop high blood pressure in the future. About *90 percent* of Americans will develop hypertension (a blood pressure higher than 140/90) at some point in their lives. Shocking, we know! High blood pressure affects one in three adults—that's 72 million Americans! Prehypertension affects another 69 million Americans, and the biggest culprit for developing prehypertension is salt intake.

> **"What's in a Number?"**
>
> Normal blood pressure is 120/80. Here's what those numbers mean:
>
> **Systolic blood pressure** is the pressure against the artery walls when the heart contracts to pump blood to the body. It is the first of the two numbers, and the higher of the two. Optimal systolic blood pressure is below 120. A systolic pressure between 120 and 139 is considered prehypertension, and over 140 is hypertension.
>
> **Diastolic blood pressure** is the pressure that exists against the walls of the arteries when the heart relaxes between beats. It is the second and lower of the two numbers. Optimal diastolic blood pressure is 80 or below. A diastolic pressure between 80 and 89 is considered prehypertension, and 90 or above is hypertension.

People with prehypertension are two and a half times more likely to develop cardiovascular disease over the following twelve years than people with normal blood pressure. People with prehypertension also have double the risk of dying from cardiovascular disease than people with normal blood pressure.

> A study published in the *British Medical Journal* found that when people who had **prehypertension** or early-stage high blood pressure reduced their sodium intake by 25 to 35 percent, they lowered their risk of cardiovascular problems by 25 percent and their risk of death by 20 percent for up to fifteen years.

The average American consumes 3,000 to 5,000 milligrams of sodium a day. If you cut out 25 to 30 percent of your intake you would just barely reach the maximum amount of sodium you *should* be consuming. And that could save your life. (Hopefully those white crystals are becoming a little less tempting.)

According to the Institute of Medicine, the adequate intake of sodium for people 19 to 50 years old is 1,500 milligrams (3.8 grams of salt) per day, the amount it takes to replace the average amount lost in a day from sweat, tears, and other bodily processes. The American Heart Association, the USDA, and the 2005 Dietary Guidelines for Americans all recommend consuming less than 2,300 milligrams of sodium per day (about 5 grams of salt), which is equivalent to about 1 teaspoon of salt. So the average American actually consumes *twice the recommended amount!* It may not sound like a big difference, but it's enough to influence your health. And it's a far cry from the 600 to 750 milligrams of sodium that our ancestors took in. The human body is not biologically designed to handle as much salt as we now consume, which is why excess salt is such a health concern.

> **Hypertension** is the leading cause of cardiovascular disease (CVD). It affects 1 billion people worldwide and is the most common reason for visits to doctor's offices and the primary reason for prescription drug use.

Weight-Saving SWAP

Think You Can't Drop the Salt?
Try These Sodium-Saving Swaps

• Leave that tablespoon of butter off your daily morning toast and use I Can't Believe It's Not Butter! spray instead; *you'll save almost 10.5 pounds in a year and 13 days' worth of sodium.*

• Dump that biscuit with 12 grams of fat and 750 milligrams of sodium and have a whole wheat dinner roll instead. *Do this twice a week and save three pounds per year and 26 days' worth of sodium.*

• Switch your morning bowl of Special K (330 milligrams of sodium) to a bowl of oatmeal with fresh blueberries (0 milligrams of sodium) three days a week *and save 7 days' worth of sodium a year.*

• Swap Wolfgang Puck's All Natural Uncured Pepperoni Pizza (1,110 calories, 2,370 milligrams of sodium, 51 grams of fat) for South Beach Diet Harvest Wheat Crust Grilled Chicken & Vegetables Pizza (330 calories, 600 milligrams of sodium, and 10 grams of fat); or Lean Cuisine Deep Dish Margherita Pizza (340 calories, 540 milligrams of sodium, and 9 grams of fat); or Healthy Choice Gourmet Supreme Pizza (360 calories, 460 milligrams of sodium, and 4 grams of fat).

• Want to be five pounds lighter tomorrow? Swap your Chinese restaurant General Tso's Chicken (1,300 calories, 3,200 milligrams of sodium, and 11 grams of saturated fat) for one cup of chicken and snow peas, one cup of brown rice, and a side of steamed broccoli (501 calories, 379 milligrams of sodium, and 0.5 grams of saturated fat).

• Want another swap to make you five pounds lighter the next morning? Swap your miso soup, crunchy shrimp roll, tempura roll, and spicy salmon = **GRAND TOTAL: 2,019 CALORIES; 4,052 MILLIGRAMS OF SODIUM** for: 2 cups unsalted edamame with pods, salmon with wasabi, 1 tablespoon low-sodium soy sauce on the side, and steamed veggies with one half cup of brown rice = **GRAND TOTAL: 400 CALORIES, 639 MILLIGRAMS OF SODIUM.** You'll save 1,619 calories and 3,413 milligrams of sodium. *Do this once a week and you'll save 24 pounds and 77 days of sodium a year!*

Calcium Loss and Osteoporosis

If you take the time to work out and perform weight-bearing exercises a few days a week to keep your bones strong, all of your hard work could be undermined by eating too much salty food. Unbelievable, but true. Studies show that postmenopausal women with a high-salt diet lose more bone minerals than other women of the same age, putting them at higher risk of osteoporosis. And don't think that just because you haven't yet gone through menopause you can eat all the salt you want. The typical American diet contains so much sodium that it results in a lack of calcium absorption from the food you eat—*in any age group*. Considering that most Americans don't meet the minimum daily calcium requirements, less calcium absorption spells trouble and it results in weaker bones over time. The two minerals, sodium and calcium, compete to be reabsorbed in the kidneys, and when more sodium than calcium is in the body, the sodium wins entry into the kidneys. Since there is a lot more sodium than calcium in our food, it is no surprise that calcium loses out most of the time. It has been found that for every 2,300 milligrams of sodium you take in, you lose about 40 milligrams of calcium. Considering that the average American takes in about 4,000 milligrams of sodium per day, we're talking about a calcium loss of almost 80 milligrams a day. The recommended amount of calcium is 1,000 milligrams a day for adult men and women (up until the age of 50), and the average intake is only 737 milligrams a day. You probably already don't get what you need,

> Need another reason to cut back on your salt even if you're young? It's not just adults anymore. Thanks to poor dietary habits—including eating lots of processed foods—and lack of exercise (both of which also impact the obesity epidemic), there has been a significant increase in the percentage of young adults, age eighteen and older, who have high blood pressure.

never mind the excess you lose from your sodium intake. The good news is we can help both problems with effective exercises and our salt-slashing lifestyle plan.

So get ready to improve your blood pressure, reduce your risk of heart disease, and beat the battle of the bulge—and bloat—for good.

Chapter 2

Your Jumpstart to Skinny: Meet the Green Light Foods— Slimmers, Anti-Bloaters, and Flushers

The Jumpstart Plan is phase 1 of your slimming plan. This is not only a cutthroat, no-bloat phase, but a weight-loss jumpstart, too. It will also be your fallback plan—any time that you are feeling bloated, chunky, or sluggish, or if you need to get in shape fast, you can repeat this phase. The Jumpstart Plan is stricter than the Maintenance Plan, which you'll follow after completing the Jumpstart Plan. Some super-dedicated followers may want to continue this hard-core plan even when the Jumpstart phase ends; if this is your style, go for it. However, since the Jumpstart Plan is rigorous, it may be too challenging to follow for an extended length of time. During this phase you may lose 10 pounds or more from fat loss, fluid shifts, and release of the bloat.* For the calorie-conscious, the Jumpstart Plan is about 1,200 calories for

_____

*For optimal results, it's important to begin exercise during this phase. See chapter 9 for some ideas._

women and about 1,400 calories for men with two snacks allowed each day. To see sample Jumpstart Meal Plans, turn to page 47.

The Green Light Foods: Your Weight-Loss Allies

The Green Light foods—Slimmers, Flushers, and Anti-Bloaters—are the keys to your lean, bloat-free life. Focus on eating them, and you will watch the pounds melt off and stay off. By eating these foods only, you'll avoid the biggest weight loss saboteurs—the Pluggers, Flabbers, Bloaters, and Chubbers that inflate your body and inevitably deflate your ego.

SLIMMERS

There are four different kinds of Slimmers—Carbohydrate Slimmers, Protein Slimmers, Mono Slimmers, and Beverage Slimmers.

"Carbohydrate Slimmers" (List A in Appendix I) are primarily whole grains, foods like whole-grain breads, whole-grain pasta, whole-grain tortillas, brown rice, oatmeal, and fruits, and they should be included at every meal. Carbohydrate Slimmers provide your body with energy and are packed with the important vitamins that help turn food into usable energy. Unlike white bread and other highly processed and refined carbohydrates, they aren't stripped of their fiber and valuable nutrients, so the energy they provide is long-lasting without causing sugar highs or crashes. They'll help to slim you down *and* de-bloat you. You'll feel fueled and won't crave excess food for a pick-me-up. And you'll have the energy that you need to exercise. What's more, the fiber will help keep you feeling full longer and help prevent constipation—and, of course, the unsightly gut bulges that come with it.

"Protein Slimmers" (List B in Appendix I), such as fish, shrimp, eggs, chicken breast, low-fat/nonfat dairy products, tofu, and beans, help to build and repair calorie-blasting muscle tissue and keep your muscles firm and toned. They take longer to digest than Carbohydrate Slimmers and should be included at each meal as they help to extend the energy boost from the carbohydrates and increase satiety. So remember: For the best energy-revving, fat-blasting potential, every meal should contain a Carbohydrate Slimmer and a Protein Slimmer. *Carbohydrates and protein at every meal?!* Who ever said losing weight couldn't be fun?

"Mono Slimmers" (List C in Appendix I) are foods that contain significant amounts of healthy monounsaturated fats, such as olive oil, almonds, pistachios, sunflower seeds, walnuts, and avocados, that slow digestion, prolong fullness, and create more sustained energy. Plus, they help to keep your arteries unclogged and flexible, allowing nutrients and oxygen to flow swiftly, energizing your muscles and rejuvenating your skin. Mono Slimmers are typically high in the antioxidant vitamin E, which helps keep inflammation at bay, lending a hand in the antiaging department. These "miracle" workers can truly transform your body, specifically targeting dangerous and hard-to-lose belly fat in a way that no other nutrient can. The key is to ditch foods that are refined, full of sugar, and high in artery-clogging saturated and trans fats and replace them with Mono Slimmers. Despite their benefits, Mono Slimmers are high in calories, so their portion sizes are small. Surprisingly, 1 tablespoon of olive oil is a whopping 120 calories, so take heed or you will negate their slimming effects.

"Beverage Slimmers" include water and tea, ideally green, black, or oolong, which you'll have with meals and snacks. Both beverages offer a myriad of health, weight, and anti-bloating

> **Antioxidants: A-C-E Your Way to Stellar Health**
>
> **Vitamin A** is essential for healthy skin, fighting infections and boosting immunity, and for nighttime vision. Where to get it: low-fat and nonfat cheese, eggs, oily fish (such as mackerel), fat-free and 1% milk, fortified trans-free margarine, and low-fat and nonfat yogurt.
>
> **Vitamin C**: Boosts immunity and protects against cardiovascular disease, prenatal health problems, eye disease, and even skin wrinkling. Where to get it: fruits and vegetables.
>
> **Vitamin E**: Protects cell membranes, including skin cells, against damage. Where to get it: plant oils such as soy and corn; the best choices are canola and olive oil. Other good sources include nuts and seeds, and wheat germ.

benefits. They fill your stomach without calories, and they keep you hydrated, which helps your body to function at its best. Every process in the body relies on water; without enough, all body functions suffer, including your energy level and metabolism. While it seems counterintuitive to drink water or tea when you're feeling waterlogged, they help beat the bloat by restoring sodium balance and flushing out salt and the excess water it attracts. Plus, they help stimulate your intestinal tract, preventing constipation. They are especially important when you increase the fiber in your diet, which you will be doing in this plan, because the liquids help to flush the fiber out of your body. An added bonus? Water and tea improve the appearance of wrinkles by filling skin cells and flushing toxins, producing a more youthful and radiant glow.

FLUSHERS AND ANTI-BLOATERS

"**Flushers**" and "**Anti-Bloaters**" (List D in Appendix I) include fruits and nonstarchy vegetables, such as blueberries, oranges, grapefruit, pineapple, strawberries, cantaloupe, watermelon, broccoli, celery, cucumbers, lettuce, red peppers, and spinach. In addition to including a Carbohydrate Slimmer and a Protein Slimmer at each meal, you will round out at least two of your three daily meals with vegetables and/or fruits from the Flushers and Anti-Bloaters list. Both women and men will limit fruits to two a day. You'll often have more than one Flusher or Anti-Bloater per meal in order to meet your required five to nine servings of vegetables. This will help fill you up without filling you out! Vegetables are super-low in calories, yet filling, thanks to their high water content and fiber.

Consuming adequate Flushers and Anti-Bloaters will help you achieve the minimum 25 grams (for women) or 38 grams (for men) of fiber that are necessary daily for good health. (*Note: Women and men over fifty should get 21 and 30 grams, respectively.*)

Slimmers, Flushers, and Anti-Bloaters are wholesome, nutrient-rich foods that are low in sodium and fat. They each contain special nutrients to keep you bloat-free and energized while working synergistically to contribute uniquely to your weight loss. Read on and we will show you how to combine them to optimize your slim-down process.

How to Build Your Meals on the Jumpstart Plan

Research shows that eating small, frequent meals throughout the day is beneficial to a speedy metabolism and losing weight. Surprisingly, skipping meals leads to weight gain.

Your goal should be to have a "mini-meal" every three to five hours. Although our menus list three main meals and two snacks, you might better think of these as five "mini-meals" spaced every three to five hours. This spacing provides a constant source of fuel for your body so that it doesn't need to conserve calories and fat for energy. You won't feel ravenous, so you won't have the binges that often accompany hunger. A continuous supply of energy prevents peaks and valleys in both your energy level and your mood.

You'll create a Jumpstart meal by choosing one food from List A, List B, and List D (see Table 1). You can also choose an option from List C *once a day* and up to four condiment "Freebies." Since you're detoxing your body of excess sodium, your goal is to keep your daily sodium intake to 1,500 milligrams. Note that Table 2 lists only the general guidelines for food categories; specific brand names are included in the lists in Appendix I. After just a little practice, it's easy to put together a slimming meal, but if you'd prefer not to bother with counting foods, you can follow the menus on page 47. If you don't want to measure your food, the Rule of Hand will help keep portions in check (see page 88), but remember that your weight-loss results may be less dramatic if you choose not to follow the specific serving sizes.

Table 1: Jumpstart Plan Daily Servings

	Servings per Day (Women)	Servings per Day (Men)
Carbohydrate Slimmers (List A Foods)	4	5
Protein Slimmers (List B Foods)	5 (at least 2 from Dairy)	6.5 (at least 2 from Dairy)
Mono Slimmers (List C Foods)	1	1
Flushers/Anti-Bloaters (List D Foods)	5–9 Vegetables (Work your way up to 9.) 2 Fruits	5–10 Vegetables (Work your way up to 9 or 10.) 2 Fruits
Beverage Slimmers (Water or Tea)	8+ (See page 41 for number of servings based on your weight.)	8+ (See page 41 for number of servings based on your weight.)
Freebies	4	4

Table 2: Slimmer Servings

Jumpstart Food	Sodium Limit 1,500 mg a day	Jumpstart Slimmer Serving Qualifications	Count Each Serving As
CARBOHYDRATE SLIMMERS (List A Foods)			
Bread (whole grains only): wraps, pita, English muffins, other whole grains like brown rice and popcorn	≤110 mg sodium per serving	≤120 calories ≥2 grams fiber	1 Carbohydrate Slimmer
	≤175 mg sodium per serving	121–150 calories ≥2 grams fiber	1.5 Carbohydrate Slimmers
	≤200 mg sodium per serving	151–200 calories ≥2 grams fiber	2 Carbohydrate Slimmers

Jumpstart Food	Sodium Limit 1,500 mg a day	Jumpstart Slimmer Serving Qualifications	Count Each Serving As
CARBOHYDRATE SLIMMERS (List A Foods) *continued*			
Whole Grain Pasta	≤5 mg sodium per serving	≤120 calories ≥2 grams fiber	1 Carbohydrate Slimmer
Cereal: whole grains only—first ingredient reads "whole"	≤110 mg sodium per serving	≤120 calories ≤8 grams sugar ≥5 grams fiber (≥3 grams fiber if hot cereal)	1 Carbohydrate Slimmer
	≤175 mg sodium per serving	121–150 calories ≤12 grams sugar ≥5 grams fiber (≥3 grams fiber if hot cereal)	1.5 Carbohydrate Slimmers
	≤220 mg sodium per serving	151–200 calories ≤16 grams sugar ≥5 grams fiber (≥3 grams fiber if hot cereal)	2 Carbohydrate Slimmers
Starchy Vegetables, Starchy Tomato Sauce, Beans, fresh or canned/processed (ideally "no salt added" or "low-sodium") *(Note: You can count beans as a Carbohydrate Slimmer or a Protein Slimmer)*	≤140 mg sodium per serving	50–100 calories (starchy veggies and starchy tomato sauces) ½ cup serving for beans	1 Carbohydrate Slimmer
PROTEIN SLIMMERS (List B Foods)			
Cheese, Milk (and Soy Milk), and Other Dairy Products	≤ 240 mg sodium per serving Cottage cheese: ≤ 380 mg sodium, limit to one ½-cup serving per day	≤3 grams fat per serving Yogurt: ≤100 calories, ≤12 grams of sugar, ≥ 5 grams protein, ≥20% DV calcium per 6-ounce serving; ≥10% per 6-ounce Greek yogurt; Soy Milk: ≤100 calories per serving	1 Protein Slimmer (Dairy serving)

Jumpstart Food	Sodium Limit 1,500 mg a day	Jumpstart Slimmer Serving Qualifications	Count Each Serving As
PROTEIN SLIMMERS (List B Foods) *continued*			
Meat, Fish, Poultry, Tofu, Tempeh	≤140 mg sodium per 2-ounce serving of single, raw ingredient	Choose only skinless poultry breast, beef round or loin, or pork tenderloin (limit beef and pork to twice a week); fish and canned chicken (only "low-sodium" and "no salt added," canned in water varieties)	1 Protein Slimmer
Shellfish Clams, Oysters, Scallops, Shrimp, Squid (aka Calamari)	≤140 mg sodium per 2-ounce serving of single, raw ingredient	Limit to twice a week	1 Protein Slimmer
Beans: dried, canned/processed (ideally "no salt added" or "low-sodium") (Note: You can count beans as a Carbohydrate Slimmer or a Protein Slimmer)	≤140 mg sodium per serving	Beans (≤ 140 mg per ½-cup serving) and those that specify "no salt added" or "low-sodium"	1 Protein Slimmer
Deli Meats	≤480 mg sodium per 2-ounce serving	Low-sodium varieties only	1 Protein Slimmer
MONO SLIMMERS (List C Foods)			
Fats, Oils, Spreads	≤140 mg sodium per serving	Limit to 100-calorie portions Monounsaturated fats only (no butter)	1 Mono Slimmer

Jumpstart Food	Sodium Limit 1,500 mg a day	Jumpstart Slimmer Serving Qualifications	Count Each Serving As
MONO SLIMMERS (List C Foods) *continued*			
Seeds, Nuts, Nut Butters, Sauces, Hummus	≤240 mg sodium per serving Hummus: <150 mg sodium per 3 tablespoons	Limit to 100-calorie servings Unsalted nuts, nut butters only If unable to find unsalted hummus, stick to a 3-tablespoon serving to keep sodium in check	1 Mono Slimmer (Nuts serving)
FLUSHERS AND ANTI-BLOATERS (List D Foods)			
Non-Starchy Vegetables, Fruits, Non-Starchy Tomato Sauce: fresh or canned/processed ("no salt added" or "low-sodium" only)	≤140 mg sodium per serving	≤50 calories for vegetables and tomato sauce ≤100 calories for fresh fruits and fruits canned in own juice only (no syrup) Canned pumpkin: any variety allowed	1 Flusher/ Anti-Bloater
CONDIMENTS			
Freebies	≤20 mg sodium per serving	≤10 calories	1 Freebie
	≤40 mg sodium per serving	≤20–25 calories	2 Freebies
BEVERAGES			
Tea and Water	≤10 mg sodium per 8-ounce serving	Tea (preferably green, black, or oolong with no added sugar) (5 of your beverage servings per day should be tea)	1 Beverage Slimmer

Green Light Foods: The Details

In the rest of this chapter we'll give you the "nitty-gritty" of the Green Light foods that will make up your Jumpstart Plan. If you don't like to count foods or if you can't be bothered with specifics, you can jump straight to the menus or take a peek at the Jumpstart food lists and choose foods from there. Just make sure to avoid the foods we list as Red Light foods (see page 143).

The Nitty-Gritty of the Carbohydrate Slimmers

	Servings per Day (Women)	Servings per Day (Men)
Carbohydrate Slimmers (List A Foods)	4	5

Each Carbohydrate Slimmer serving contains roughly 100 calories, and during the Jumpstart phase, 110 milligrams or less of sodium. One serving is equal to ½ cup of cooked whole-grain cereal, brown rice, or pasta; a slice of whole-wheat bread; ½ whole-grain English muffin; 1 cup dry cereal; 5 crackers; or a small tortilla (4-inch) or pancake (3-inch). Each Carbohydrate Slimmer food must also meet the other requirements listed in Table 2 (such as the sugar or fat limits given for specific foods). At each meal you will include a Carbohydrate Slimmer serving (for a total of 4 per day for women, 5 per day for men).

Items in the "Starchy Veggie" category in List A, such as potatoes and corn, are technically considered vegetables but are starchy (or higher in calories) and are more similar to Carbohydrate Slimmers because they provide a significant amount of energy. Count them as Carbohydrate Slimmers. Unlike cooked whole grains, a serving size of these starchy veggies varies depending on the item. (See List A in Appendix I for specific serving sizes.)

Some items can be considered either a Carbohydrate Slimmer or a Protein Slimmer and are noted as such in Table 2. You can eat these foods alone for a snack, without having to combine them with other foods.

Our extensive List A includes only some of the many Jumpstart Carbohydrate Slimmer foods available—companies are continuously introducing new products or revamping existing ones to meet your slimming needs. Breads that didn't qualify yesterday may already have been reformulated to help in your weight-loss crusade. If you don't see your favorites on List A, they may still qualify as Carbohydrate Slimmers, as long as they're whole grain or have only a trivial amount of refined grain and fit the other slimming criteria in Table 2.

Remember, you normally should get no more than 2,300 milligrams of sodium per day, and on the Jumpstart Plan, as you detoxify your salt-saturated cells, you should get 1,500 milligrams or less. A typical slice of whole-grain bread has 177 milligrams of sodium, while a serving of brown rice or sweet potato has virtually no sodium. Even when you stick to breads that qualify as Jumpstart foods, (limited to 110 milligrams of sodium per serving), if you eat only bread for all of your Carbohydrate Slimmers servings, the sodium will add up fast (550 milligrams for men's five daily servings, and 440 milligrams for women's four). That's before you add any protein, dairy, or condiments. Avoid the "bread trap" by choosing from many of the lower-sodium options included in List A.

WHOLE-GRAIN BREADS, TORTILLAS, ENGLISH MUFFINS, AND PITAS

Whole-grain breads help you feel satisfied and make you feel like you're definitely *not* on a diet since you can eat bread! *Woo-hoo!* Unbelievably, you can eat a sandwich and be bloat-free—even in this strict phase. Make sure the first item on the label's ingredient list is the word "*whole.*" As long as the word *whole* is before the grain, whether the grain is wheat, rye, oats, or something else, you will get a wholesome grain that will help to fight cancer, heart disease, and diabetes. Seeing the word "*whole*" will ensure that your bread has

Nutrition Twins FAVORITE

Alvarado Street Bakery No Salt! Sprouted Multi-Grain Bread and Ezekiel 4:9 Organic Sprouted Whole Grain Sesame Bread

Encouraging news for those fearful of trying "no salt added" bread: Our clients tell us after a week or two they don't even notice they're not eating the regular variety. However, they do notice they're much less bloated than usual. An added bonus: many people find that although they enjoy the no-salt bread, they are less likely to overeat it.

the good stuff to keep you satisfied and lean. It also ensures fiber is naturally present to flush you out. Look for low-sodium options to make your life easier, since the sodium will be even lower than our 110-milligram requirement. Whole-grain crackers with less sodium, such as Ryvita Crispbread, also fit into this category.

WHOLE-WHEAT PASTA, BUCKWHEAT PASTA, BROWN RICE, AND QUINOA

Yes, you can eat rice and pasta while losing fat and beating the bloat. Just remember: Don't add salt to the water during cooking. Omit the salt and use herbs such as basil, oregano, parsley, and pepper to flavor them instead, or use an Italian seasoning blend. Always use garlic powder or onion powder instead of their salt forms. By adding salt, Slimmers like quinoa and rice instantly become Bloaters.

 For a slimming surprise, try buckwheat noodles instead of whole-wheat pasta. Buckwheat is hearty, high in fiber, and unlike most carbs, it contains protein so it's satiating and therefore harder to overeat than the regular stuff. Plus, it's loaded with magnesium, which helps relax blood vessels and improve blood flow and nutrient delivery while lowering blood pressure—the perfect combination for a healthy cardiovascular system, a trim, bloat-free body, and ageless skin.

WHOLE-GRAIN CEREALS

Bran cereals and other whole-grain cold and hot cereals, such as Kashi Heart to Heart and oatmeal, are Carbohydrate Slimmers that beat the bloat caused by constipation, serving as nature's "Liquid-Plumr." They provide the perfect start to your day by giving you energy to keep you active and lean. The best cold cereals are whole grain ("*whole*" must appear as the first word before the grain in the ingredient list), high in fiber, and low in sugar, salt, and fat. Good sources of whole grains include oats, oat bran, corn bran, wheat bran, Muesli, and low-fat granola. Be careful with granola as it may contain a lot of added sugar—you want no more than 8 grams of sugar per serving.

You'll find some of the most popular cereals on List A. Don't see your favorite cold cereal? Just make sure it's made from a whole grain and that it fits the criteria for a Carbohydrate Slimmer given in Table 2 at the beginning of this chapter. Don't be fooled—Corn Flakes, Smart Start, and Special K *aren't* 100 percent whole-grain cereals. They lack nutrients and fiber—and they're pretty high in salt, too. Even worse? They make you constipated and bloated.

Oatmeal has one of the highest satiety rankings of any food. This means it fills you up and keeps you satisfied so that hunger doesn't get the best of you. Unlike many carbohydrates, oats—even the instant kind—digest slowly. This

> **Nutrition Twins FAVORITE**
>
> Arrowhead Hills Steel Cut Oats and Quaker Quick Oats

means they cause a more gradual and long-lasting energy and blood sugar boost. All oats are healthful, but the steel-cut and rolled varieties (which are minimally processed) have up to 5 grams of fiber per serving, making them the most filling choice. Instant oats contain 3 to 4 grams of fiber per serving, so they are also healthy options. During this Jumpstart phase, stick to old-fashioned rolled, steel-cut, or instant plain oatmeal to keep the sodium levels low. If you must eat a flavored variety of oatmeal, try Quaker Take Heart. (It has 160 calories, so you'll count it as 2 Carbohydrate Slimmers servings.) Quaker does a great job of keeping the sodium to 110 milligrams, the sugar to 9 grams, and the fiber at 5 to 6 grams—four of which are cholesterol-lowering soluble fiber. Plus, it provides a healthy dose of potassium to counteract any sodium.

For best results, eat hot cereals plain. If you want your hot cereal sweetened, do it naturally by adding your own fruit.

Don't currently eat a lot of fiber? Then start with a half serving of bran cereal or other whole-grain, high-fiber cereal, so your body can adjust to the fiber.

POPCORN

Three cups of air-popped popcorn count as just 1 Carbohydrate Slimmer serving as long as you don't prepare it with oil and you don't add butter or salt! Try jazzing it up with a little cinnamon, I Can't Believe It's Not Butter! *spray* (not the spread), or a *sprinkle* of grated Parmesan. Check the nutrition facts for your favorite brand—it will count as a Carbohydrate Slimmer if a serving has 120 calories or less and less than 110 milligrams of sodium.

CORN, PEAS, POTATOES, WINTER SQUASH, BUTTERNUT SQUASH, AND EDAMAME BEANS

Choose these fresh or frozen, not canned. These veggies are high in fiber like other vegetables, but they are starchier, so they provide a good source of sustained energy. Their fiber content helps provide an even longer-lasting satiety and energy boost. Packed with potassium, they flush toxins and waste (and bloat!) out of your body. Their antioxidants keep skin firm and youthful.

You can think of potatoes as anti-bloating sculpters. Thanks to kukoamines and potassium, potatoes help lower blood pressure. They'll also help you kick constipation if you eat the fibrous skin. Sweet potatoes boast beta-carotene, an antioxidant that heals the body and fights aging. Of course, you'll need to nix French fries and the butter and sour cream as a topping for your spud. Top your potatoes instead with roasted garlic or garlic powder, I Can't Believe It's Not Butter! *spray*, and a spritz of lemon, and you won't ever miss the butter.

One half cup of edamame with pods equals 1 Carbohydrate Slimmer serving. Try this great restaurant appetizer at home—it also contains satiating protein and plenty of fiber to help unplug you.

TOMATO SAUCE ("LOW-SODIUM" OR "NO SALT ADDED")

Tomato sauces with 50 to 100 calories per ½ cup serving are considered "starchy" and provide decent amounts of energy, like starchy veggies. Count each ½ cup as 1 Carbohydrate Slimmer serving. (Those with less than 50 calories per ½ cup serving are Flushers/Anti-Bloaters. See List D in Appendix I for specific food listings.)

The Nitty-Gritty of Protein Slimmers

	Servings per Day (Women)	Servings per Day (Men)
Protein Slimmers (List B Foods)	5 (at least 2 from Dairy)	6.5 (at least 2 from Dairy)

A Protein Slimmer serving is equal to 2 ounces of very lean meat, fish, or poultry; ½ cup tofu or cooked dried beans, split peas, or lentils; 4 level tablespoons of hummus; 1 egg or 4 egg whites; 1 cup milk or calcium-fortified soy milk; ¾ cup nonfat or low-fat yogurt; 1 ounce nonfat or low-fat cheese (typically one thin slice of cheese); ¼ cup nonfat or low-fat shredded cheese; or ½ cup nonfat or low-fat cottage cheese.

At least two calcium-rich foods, such as nonfat or low-fat dairy products, should contribute to your Protein Slimmer allotment. These dairy products, despite having sodium, fill you up, counteract the effects of bloating, and help to lower your blood pressure. In fact, they'll skim inches off your waist and points off your blood pressure as they're satiating you. (You'll eat less, which will help you avoid packing on the pounds.) Plus, they give you a big calcium boost, and eating a diet with adequate calcium (1,000 to 1,300 milligrams per day) results in lower body weights and less body fat. As with Carbohydrate Slimmers, if you are not one to measure your servings, see page 88 to learn the portion sizes using the Rule of Hand.

If you are losing weight too quickly (more than 10 pounds in a week) or feeling ravenous, you can add either 1 Carbohydrate Slimmer or 1 Protein Slimmer serving each day.

LEGUMES (BEANS)

Packed with iron, folic acid, potassium, and fiber, beans (excluding green or wax beans) contain what most of us don't get enough of. Plus, much of their fiber is soluble, which mops up cholesterol in your blood and lowers it. Less cholesterol means fewer plaques and less disease, so your arteries and blood vessels are more pliant and flexible and more efficient at delivering fat-burning oxygen throughout the body. What's more, beans are packed with antioxidants to revitalize your skin, and their carbohydrate/protein combo energizes every organ in your body. They're noted in List B so you will remember that you can count ½ cup as 1 Carbohydrate Slimmer *or* 1 Protein Slimmer serving. Since beans contain both carbohydrates and protein, you can eat these as a snack without combining them with another food. So munch on edamame as a snack for both energizing carbs and satiating protein.

Lentils and split peas are less gas-forming than other legumes. Plus, they're bona fide belly flatteners since they're high in protein and soluble fiber—both of which help to stabilize blood sugar levels. Eating them prevents insulin spikes that cause your body to store excess fat, especially in the abdominal area.

For most people, beans help build a trimmer, slimmer body. However, for others, beans create bloating and can be gaseous. If this is you, don't eat beans

Why Combine?

If you were to eat just Protein Slimmers, such as steak and eggs, you'd lack energy, and you'd feel bloated from constipation. If you were to eat just Carbohydrate Slimmers, such as salad and bread, you'd feel hungry soon after eating, and you'd have trouble maintaining lean muscle mass and a svelte body. When you combine these foods, such as in a sandwich, you get your carbohydrate (the bread), your protein (such as tuna), and your veggies (such as lettuce and tomato) all in one.

until you have completed the Jumpstart Plan. After the Jumpstart phase, what's a bloated bean-lover to do? Try "Beano." Take this nonprescription liquid or tablet immediately before consuming beans. If it works for you, problem solved! If that still doesn't work for you, start with a very small portion of beans (just a table-spoon or two) and take Beano when you eat them. Gradually increase your bean intake in the Maintenance phase to help your body adjust without symptoms. Beans are too good to miss out on.

 Eating canned beans? *Always* rinse them in cold water and drain them to save your gut in two priceless ways. You'll wash away a lot of the belly-expand-ing sodium (as much as 40 percent!) that is used in the canning process, and you'll also rinse away some potentially gas-producing properties.

SKINLESS POULTRY BREAST

To keep poultry as a healthy option, stick to the white meat and avoid the skin. Dark meat has about 15 percent more calories and 30 to 40 percent more fat than white meat. *Yikes!* Steer clear of fatty duck and beware of ground turkey and turkey burgers. Unless they are made from *breast* meat, they include the dark meat and the skin and are as fatty as regular hamburger meat. Fresh-sliced turkey or chicken breast is an ideal Protein Slimmer—keep it in the fridge to grab for a sandwich or to top a salad. If you are choosing deli-sliced poultry, choose low-sodium varieties. Avoid other deli slices—at least during the Jumpstart Plan. Ban smoked varieties; the salt will puff you up almost before it touches your lips.

Make sure your rotisserie chicken hasn't been doused with salt. Added salt is often injected, so even when you remove the skin the salt remains. Slice your unsalted rotisserie chicken (without the fattening skin, of course) as soon as you get home; it's easier to remove from the bone when it's warm. Freeze extras for later.

Unfortunately, just because a chicken label says "Natural," it doesn't mean your chicken is free from added salt. Some chickens have added sodium and water. We know—it's a disgrace. The amount of injected sodium varies. Chicken breasts can have as little as 119 milligrams of added sodium per serving (5 percent of the recommended daily maximum, which is still too much for our bloat-free minds), and turkey breasts may contain as much as 373 milligrams (16 percent of the daily maximum). Remember that 40 to 50 milligrams of sodium already occur naturally, so adding more makes this an unhealthy option.

Therefore, avoid any poultry with added ingredients.

Nutrition Twins FAVORITE

Harvestland boneless, skinless chicken breasts. They're tasty and delicious, free of additives and preservatives, and contain no antibiotics, hormones, or steroids.

Even though it costs more per pound, poultry that is free of additional sodium is available (check the label). For example, a good option is Perdue's Fit & Easy line (not the Tender & Tasty line). Choose any of their boneless, skinless breasts, ground chicken, and ground turkey breast. Most are 99 percent fat-free, and all are fresh and have no artificial additives or preservatives.

LEAN MEATS

Eating beef? Grill, broil, or bake it. Cut off the excess fat to make a lean, bloat-free Protein Slimmer option. Although 1 Protein Slimmer is 2 ounces of meat, limit beef to no more than 3 ounces (which is 1½ Protein Slimmers), twice a week to keep your heart healthy and to stave off cancer. When it comes to ground beef, don't be tricked by "lean" or "extra lean" labels with claims of "10% fat" or "90% lean." This is the percentage of fat by weight, not the *percentage of calories from fat*. If you buy ground beef that is 80 percent lean, you aren't doing yourself any favors. A whopping 300 of the 430 calories in an 80 percent lean quarter-pounder come from fat! Stay away from ground beef during the Jumpstart Phase unless you choose ground beef from the round or from the loin.

FISH

By far, fish is one of the best proteins. The omega-3 fatty acids in fish protect the heart by helping maintain a normal heart rhythm, lowering triglycerides, and making blood less "sticky." "Sticky" blood means plaques, which cling to artery walls, clogging them and increasing heart attack and stroke risk. Plus, omega-3s are anti-aging because they reduce inflammation—yes, this means they help get rid of swelling and puffy under-eye bags. They also improve insulin sensitivity, helping to build muscle and decrease belly fat. And the more muscle you have, the more calories your body burns.

A higher omega-3 diet helps beat the bloat and lower blood pressure; this may mean that fish prevent some of salt's damage. Although the fish that are highest in omega-3 fatty acids, such as salmon, herring, anchovies, oysters, sardines, whitefish, and mackerel, have the most of these benefits, their portion size is slightly smaller because they are higher in calories.

Choosing canned fish? During the Jumpstart phase, do so only if it's a "no salt added" or "low in sodium" variety. Salt your fish, and you'll make it a Bloater. Fry it, and it's a Chubber.

SHELLFISH (CLAMS, OYSTERS, SCALLOPS, AND SHRIMP ONLY), SQUID (AKA CALAMARI)

Low in calories and saturated fat, shellfish is a great source of lean protein. Although shellfish do contain a little more sodium than most fish and have higher amounts of cholesterol, it is saturated fat and excessive calories that cause trouble, and shellfish has little of either. Limit shellfish to twice a week. You'll find lobster, crab, and mussels in the Maintenance phase (chapter 6) since they are higher in sodium.

NONFAT AND LOW-FAT DAIRY

Fat-free (skim) and 1% milk, yogurt, cottage cheese, and cheese are Protein Slimmers. Generally, a serving of dairy is equal to 1 cup of milk or calcium-fortified soy milk; ¾ cup yogurt; 1 ounce cheese (typically one thin slice); ¼ cup shredded cheese; or ½ cup cottage cheese or frozen yogurt.

Nonfat and low-fat dairy products are great Slimmers because they provide the best balance of calcium, potassium, and magnesium for controlling blood pressure and combating the ill-effects of salt. In fact, fat-free and low-fat dairy products are so beneficial that they are prescribed as a primary component in the diet for someone with high blood pressure. But remember to look for low-sodium dairy products and avoid processed cheese. When choosing cottage cheese, if you don't choose low-sodium, limit your intake of it to 1 serving per day.

 Be aware that *reduced-fat* cheese is NOT *low fat.* "Reduced fat" just means that it has 25 percent less fat than the original. An ounce (about one slice) of Lorraine brand reduced-fat, low-sodium cheese still has a whopping 110 calories and 6 grams of fat, 4 of them artery clogging! This is a flab-creating, heart-clogging disaster. Always choose a "low-fat" or "nonfat" cheese over a "reduced-fat" cheese. (An exception: Cabot cheese, which reads "75% reduced fat," is much better than the usual reduced-fat cheese.)

Lower-fat and fat-free products can be higher in sodium than their full-fat counterparts: an ounce of full-fat sharp Cheddar cheese has 45 percent less sodium than an ounce of fat-free cheddar. When fat, a major vehicle for flavor, is removed, other ingredients such as sodium are often added to compensate. Even so, the tradeoff is worth it. Limit belt-bursting and damaging, artery-clogging saturated fat in your diet by enjoying low-fat and fat-free foods. You'll limit sodium in other areas instead.

Low-fat and nonfat yogurt fit the qualifications to be Protein Slimmers *or* Carbohydrate Slimmers. This means that since they have both carbohydrate and protein, you can eat yogurt on its own for a snack. Good news: whichever you choose to count it toward, you've also met one of your calcium-rich slimming choices. An added bonus? Yogurt's anti-bloating benefits are astounding. But remember, a regular, full-fat dairy product will chub you and bloat you. List B in Appendix I includes some of the acceptable dairy products in the Protein Slimmer category. Don't see your favorite yogurt? It may still qualify. See Table 2 at the beginning of this chapter to see if it meets the qualifications.

> **Nutrition Twins FAVORITE**
>
> Stonyfield Farms plain nonfat yogurt. We eat ours "slushy-style." Simply put it in the freezer for about an hour until it becomes icy. Eat it as is or blend it in a food processor to make it rich and creamy. Add 1/4 teaspoon cocoa powder. Delicious!

Although the 12 grams of sugar that you are permitted in 6 ounces of yogurt may seem like a lot, 8 of those sugar grams are there naturally. This means that the yogurt you eat during the Jumpstart phase actually has no more than 4 grams of added sugar.

Some people prefer fat-free Greek-style yogurt, which has more protein but less calcium than other yogurts. Brands such as 0% Fage Greek Yogurt and Oikos Organic Greek Yogurt (it's fat-free) taste as if they're actually full-fat! If you choose one of these types of yogurt, be sure yours has 10 percent or more of the Daily Value (DV) for calcium.

CALCIUM

As we mentioned earlier, in order to help meet your calcium requirements, you'll need at least 2 dairy servings (or calcium-rich or calcium-fortified foods) as part of your Protein Slimmers. Men, if you eat these 2 servings there's no need to take a supplement since

> **Beware of Added Fiber**
>
> Companies now add isolated fibers like inulin and polydextrose to foods such as Stonyfield Farm yogurt, Weight Watchers cereals, and Fibersure fiber supplement, claiming that they are as great as naturally occurring fibers like those found in whole grains, fruits, and vegetables. Although there isn't good evidence to support or deny this, the downside is that inulin may cause gas or other stomach distress, and a product with polydextrose may result in "a laxative effect from excessive consumption," as the package warns. Check labels and keep track of how you respond in your Food Log (see chapter 5).

Self-Diagnosed Lactose Intolerant?

Have your doctor double-check. Some people mistake irritable bowel syndrome for lactose intolerance; others think they are lactose intolerant when it is full-fat dairy that is causing bloating or flatulence. Often they can eat low-fat and nonfat dairy products and remain symptom free.

Both yogurt and kefir (a cultured dairy product similar to a yogurt drink) contain bacteria called probiotics that aid lactose digestion. Yogurt (not the frozen kind!) often doesn't produce symptoms of lactose intolerance because these bacteria help digest lactose. Plus, probiotics may reduce antibiotic-associated diarrhea and help irritable bowel syndrome and other intestinal conditions.

Luckily, everyone produces the necessary lactase enzyme which digests lactose (the sugar in milk). If you're lactose intolerant, your body simply doesn't make sufficient quantities so you don't digest milk products very effectively. You may be surprised to know that you can eat some dairy without encountering ill-effects. Although a cup of yogurt or ice cream may hurt your stomach, half may not. Everyone varies in the type and amounts of dairy products they can handle. The ideal way to discover your limit is to start with a very small portion and see if it affects you. For instance, if your milk bothers you, have a teaspoon. If this is okay, the next day try a tablespoon, and soon you'll find your limit.

If you react to lactose even in low-fat or nonfat yogurt, you can try the lactase enzyme, which is available without a prescription. Simply take it with the first bite of dairy food, and you may be able to eat dairy symptom free. If you are supersensitive to lactose, avoid it and check with a registered dietitian to ensure that you're meeting your calcium needs. Beware that small amounts of lactose may be found in many processed foods: breads and other baked goods; breakfast cereals; instant potatoes; soups; breakfast drinks; margarine; lunch meats (other than kosher ones); salad dressings; candies and other snacks; pancake mixes; biscuits; cookies; powdered meal-replacement supplements; and even "nondairy" products. If they contain whey, curds, milk by-products, dry milk solids, or nonfat dry milk powder, they've got lactose.

some studies indicate this would increase your risk of prostate cancer. We realize that while you are on the Jumpstart Plan, calories are restricted and it may be difficult to get 2 servings of dairy daily, but try your best. Women, you'll need to take 500 milligrams in calcium supplements every day. Dietary calcium requirements are high—1,000 milligrams per day for adults nineteen to fifty years old and 1,200 milligrams for those fifty and older. You would have to get 3 to 5 servings of calcium-rich foods every day to meet these requirements. Aside from dairy, foods rich in calcium include, among others, broccoli, spinach, canned salmon, and calcium-fortified juices. Look for calcium citrate or calcium carbonate supplements and split the dose up into 250 milligrams twice a day, since you can't absorb more than about 500 milligrams of calcium in one sitting from a supplement. Being on a calorie-restricted diet makes meeting calcium needs more challenging. Consult a registered dietitian if you are having problems getting adequate amounts of calcium-rich foods and don't take a calcium supplement.

Take a calcium supplement that includes magnesium as it helps to prevent constipation. Also make sure your supplement includes vitamin D to aid in calcium's absorption.

SOYBEANS AND TOFU

Soybeans are found in products such as soy milk, tempeh (which is a fermented soy cake), and tofu. Whole soy foods—those not comprised of isolated soy proteins and not processed—are a great source of protein and contain other nutrients such as fiber, B vitamins, and omega-3 fatty acids; some are fortified with calcium. Processed soy foods such as meat substitutes are not allowed on the Jumpstart Plan but will be permitted in the phase 2 Maintenance Plan.

Some studies raise concerns about soy—mainly soy isolates or other similarly processed forms of soy. Choose soy foods in the least processed form available (whole soybeans, tofu, tempeh, and products made with soy flour). *Hmmm*

… less processed? Sounds familiar—just like everything else in this plan. Soy can be a valuable source of protein in a vegetarian or vegan diet, but don't rely on it as your sole source of protein. Just because a little bit of something is good, a lot is not necessarily better.

The Nitty-Gritty of Mono Slimmers

	Servings per Day (Women)	Servings per Day (Men)
Mono Slimmers (List C Foods)	1	1

A Mono Slimmer serving contains roughly 100 calories; during the Jumpstart phase, all Mono Slimmers are virtually sodium free, with the exception of hummus, which can have up to 150 milligrams of sodium. For the most part, 1 serving is equal to 3 teaspoons of oil, 6 teaspoons (2 tablespoons) of unsalted nuts, ¼ cup avocado, or 3 level tablespoons of hummus. You can have 1 Mono Slimmer serving per day.

Mono Slimmers are like Protein Slimmers in that they take a longer time to digest and help to keep you satiated. Therefore, you can opt to have your Mono Slimmer serving in a meal to replace the Protein Slimmer, or you can have a Mono Slimmer, such as nuts, as a snack on its own.

OLIVE, CANOLA, PEANUT, SAFFLOWER, WALNUT, SUNFLOWER, SESAME, SOYBEAN, AND FLAXSEED OILS

These oils are high in monounsaturated fats, and they lower "bad" LDL cholesterol without affecting "good" HDL cholesterol. They're great alternatives to fatty, artery-clogging butter. Rich in antioxidants, they may help reduce the risk of cancer and other chronic diseases. You will need to measure these carefully because the calories add up quickly. Just pouring oil for a split second longer than intended could add an unexpected several hundred calories!

FLAXSEED

Including high-fiber flaxseed (not the oil) in your diet is a great way to stay regular and to flush out unsightly gut bulges. Flaxseed is rich in alpha linolenic acid (ALA), an omega-3 fat that is a precursor to the form of omega-3 found in fish oils—so it has anti-inflammatory properties, making it a perfect anti-ager. However, be warned: you'd have to eat a large quantity of flaxseed (and *a lot of calories*) to get the same benefits as eating a 3-ounce serving of omega-3-rich fish. Flaxseed bothers some people's stomachs, but it may be because they are not used to the high amount of fiber. Keeping a food journal (see chapter 5) will help you recognize foods that bother you.

 Whole flaxseed will pass though your body undigested. To reap nutritional benefits, grind it or buy it already ground in a vacuum-sealed package to prevent rancidity. Store ground flaxseed in a tightly sealed container in the refrigerator or freezer to prevent spoilage; once ground, flaxseed oxidizes and spoils quickly).

NUTS, SEEDS, AND THEIR BUTTERS

From almonds to pine nuts and peanut butter to tahini, these foods pack a satisfying punch. Antioxidants such as vitamin E and energy-generating B vitamins make these protein-rich, heart-healthy fats nutrient powerhouses. Choose unsalted varieties and avoid reduced-fat nut butters—surprisingly, you lose all the good stuff when they take out the fat: the Mono Slimmer benefits are removed and replaced with carbohydrates and extra salt.

Nutrition Twins FAVORITE

Unsalted pistachios. They truly are the skinny nut. Their high protein, fiber, and healthy fat combo makes them satiating, while their shells make you mindful of what you're eating. Plus, you can eat 30 of them for 100 calories!

AVOCADOS

Delicious and nutritious, the trick to gut-busting here is to eat just ¼ cup as a serving. An entire avocado could cost you 300 to 400 calories. *Yikes!*

The Nitty-Gritty of Flushers and Anti-Bloaters

	Servings per Day (Women)	Servings per Day (Men)
Flushers and Anti-Bloaters (List D Foods)	5–9 Vegetables (Work your way up to 9) 2 Fruits	5–10 Vegetables (Work your way up to 9 or 10) 2 Fruits

For the most part, a serving of vegetables is equal to 1 cup raw vegetables, 1 cup green leafy vegetables (such as lettuce), ½ cup steamed veggies, or ¾ cup vegetable juice. For fruits, a serving is usually equal to a piece of fruit or ½ cup berries or cut fruit. Here are a few fruit examples, including some exceptions to the above serving sizes. You'll find a more extensive listing of Flushers and Anti-Bloaters in List D in Appendix I.

Apple, 1 small

Applesauce, unsweetened, ½ cup

Apricots, 4

Bananas, 1 small or ½ large

Blackberries, ½ cup

Cantaloupe, ½ whole or 1 cup cubed

Cherries, ¾ cup

Grapefruit, 1 small or ½ large

Grapes, 20

Mango, 1 small, ½ large

Nectarine, 1 large

Orange, 1 large

Pineapple chunks, ¾ cup

Raisins, 3 tablespoons

Strawberries, ½ cup sliced or 1 cup whole

Fiber takes up room in your stomach, making you less hungry, so you eat less. The fiber and antioxidants found in Flushers and Anti-Bloaters provide a huge contribution to a healthy immune system—they decrease inflammation and reduce the risk of diseases such as heart disease, cancer, diabetes, and obesity. More great news—since inflammation is also linked to aging, Flushers and Anti-Bloaters will help you say, "Good-bye, wrinkles!" Plus, fiber aids a healthy digestive system.

We realize that many people complain that fiber gives them gas, which is anything but sexy. However, this usually lessens as your body adjusts to the new, appropriate amount of fiber. This plan helps you add fiber gradually, so you'll have minimal intestinal issues, if any. Plus, since fruits and vegetables are low in calories, high in fiber, and loaded with nutrients and powerful antioxidants that fight disease, they're the weight-loss secret weapon. They fill you up without puffing you out. Now that's sexy. They are naturally rich in water and potassium and low in salt—the ideal and magical anti-bloat formula that helps to restore your body's sodium balance. Eat them with each meal to relieve discomfort, bloating, and unsightly gut bulges due to constipation.

Although you can often use Flushers and Anti-Bloaters interchangeably, there are times when you will want to consume each to work to your advantage. If you are feeling constipated or bloated due to salt and water retention, it's time to pay attention to which fruits and veggies you choose. For example, if you are on an irregular schedule due to traveling and you are feeling constipated, choose vegetables and fruits that are Flushers, such as broccoli, mustard greens, pears, and apples. On the other hand, if you have splurged at a party and overindulged in salty foods, load up on Anti-Bloaters, such as asparagus, cucumbers, kale, and cantaloupe to quickly rid your body of bloat.

FRUIT

Fruits are low in calories, and most are fat free. When you eat fruits, the sugars arrive in the body packaged with fiber, large quantities of water, and many critical vitamins and minerals. In contrast, refined sugars, such as those found in candy, enter your body in a concentrated form, spiking your blood sugar and providing virtually no nutrients. Your body responds to the high dose of sugar by trying to dilute it with water. This causes you to retain water in your gut, which leads to that bloated feeling.

Fruits are a good source of wholesome, energy-providing carbohydrates; you can use one of your two fruit servings instead of a Carbohydrate Slimmer in your meal. Combine it with a Protein Slimmer and ideally with an additional Flusher for a complete meal. You can do this to save a Carbohydrate Slimmer serving when you want to have additional servings at another meal. Or, if you choose to have more than 2 daily fruit servings, the extra piece of fruit can *replace* one of your Carbohydrate Slimmer servings.

Nutrition Twins **FAVORITE**

Sunsweet Ones Dried Plums. Whenever you're feeling a little constipated or simply want to have a delicious burst of energy-boosting antioxidants, these are ideal. They're individually packaged and just 25 calories each. Toss some in your gym bag, purse, car, or suitcase. We carry them with us when we travel—a time when it's often hard to get enough fiber to be regular. These work wonders and they prevent us from craving other sweet treats.

VEGETABLES

As you know, vegetables are low-calorie, fiber-filled, and nutrient-packed, so they're perfect for anyone who wants to lose weight. They should be a component of at least two out of your three main meals each day. One of the best things about vegetables is that they contain carbohydrates, so they provide energy. And thanks to their fiber, vegetables really do fill you up. With the exception of starchy vegetables (peas, potatoes, corn, and winter and butternut squash), all vegetables can be eaten freely throughout the day without restriction. (Note: These starchy vegetables are still healthy carbohydrates, but their portion sizes must be limited, and they are counted as Carbohydrate Slimmers.) When it comes to losing body fat, vegetables are essential. Consider vegetables your "lucky charm" that you must have at lunch and dinner and as snacks. In fact, if you finish eating a meal or a snack and still feel hungry, fill up on raw or cooked vegetables.

Although you eventually want to aim for 9 vegetable servings per day in addition to 2 fruit servings, don't suddenly increase the amount of vegetables that you eat, or you may get an upset stomach with flatulence, abdominal pain, and diarrhea. Add vegetables gradually. Start by adding ¼ cup more than you typically eat at each meal; add another ¼ cup to each meal each week as you continue on to the next phase of the plan. Aim for a minimum of 1 cup of veggies with every meal. So if you aren't currently eating enough vegetables, you'll start the Jumpstart Plan with fewer vegetables than your ultimate goal, and you may feel a little bit hungrier than you will later when you can fill your stomach with more veggies. After approximately three weeks, you will be able to eat more of the foods that you are sensitive to without discomfort. Before long, you will melt body fat and look and feel slimmer than ever.

Cruciferous vegetables such as cauliflower, broccoli, cabbage, and Brussels sprouts contain glucosinalates, contributing to their cancer-protective effects. They are also known for being more gaseous, or as we say, "reactive." If these veggies cause you to "react," try cooking or steaming them to reduce their impact. Also, as mentioned above, the body adjusts to more fiber, and they tend to be less of a problem over time. They are such great Flushers that they can be a lifesaver if you're constipated. Try to include small portions (for some people this may be less than ¼ cup per meal) at two meals daily, so you adjust to them while they keep you regular and healthy.

Flushers and Anti-Bloaters: Your Extra Weight-Loss Weapons

Some fruits and vegetables are more beneficial at preventing constipation—these Flushers should be chosen any time you are feeling bloated due to constipation or any time you eat a "Plugger" (those foods that you may occasionally eat *after* the Jumpstart phase that plug you up and cause constipation). Flushers are fabulous foods such as oranges, spinach, and eggplant that are exceptionally high in fiber and flush out your colon. As an added bonus, Flushers prevent missed exercise sessions that are due to an uncomfortable, distended stomach and low energy levels.

Without Flushers, some people would always feel constipated. If this sounds familiar, you know who you are, and we feel your pain. For others who don't have

Flushers as a major part of their current diet, the key is to increase them gradually, as mentioned, so that your body has time to adjust to the fiber and all of its flushing miracles.

Anti-Bloaters are especially great at ridding your body of extra salt. While all fruits and vegetables have a high water content, Anti-Bloaters have an exceptionally high water concentration and/or an extremely high potassium concentration. Any time you are bloated due to salt overload, alcohol, or other foods, choose an Anti-Bloater. Anti-Bloaters, such as asparagus, cucumbers, bok choy, cabbage broth (if it doesn't negatively impact your digestive tract), grapefruit, tomatoes (but *not* salty tomato juice!), and watermelon, will help when you indulge in a Bloater by minimizing the damage. Note: You won't be having Bloaters during the Jumpstart phase.

Occasionally, certain Anti-Bloaters may cause intestinal distress in sensitive individuals. As you journal your diet, should you find that an Anti-Bloater is negatively effecting your intestinal tract, experiment to discover your threshold. Perhaps you can consume only small portions of the aggravating food. You simply may be unaccustomed to foods with fiber. This is common, and if it is the case, your body will adjust.

 Although parsley is an herb, not a vegetable, it is known for its anti-bloating effects, so use it to garnish potatoes, chicken, and fish. For other ideas, see "Seasoning with Slimming Spices" on page 81.

You will find the fruits and vegetables in List D in Appendix I labeled as Flushers, Anti-Bloaters, or both. Most fruits and veggies exhibit some traits of both Flushers and Anti-Bloaters. However, we label the most potent ones to help you to realize which veggies and fruits will benefit you most at times when you are constipated (labeled as Flushers) or bloated from salt overload (labeled as Anti-Bloaters). It doesn't matter whether you count the food as an Anti-Bloater or a Flusher serving, simply note that you had it and use it to your advantage to help you if you are either bloated or constipated. Those labeled Flusher/Anti-Bloater exhibit powerful anti-bloating and flushing characteristics. The fruits and vegetables are all great Flushers and Anti-Bloaters; their most powerful benefits are in parentheses.

Vegetable Flushers and Anti-Bloaters

Asparagus (Anti-Bloater)

Artichokes (Anti-Bloater)

Beets (Anti-Bloater)

Bell peppers (Flusher)

Broccoli (Flusher)

Brussels sprouts (Flusher)

Bok choy (Anti-Bloater)

Cabbage (Flusher)

Carrots (Flusher)

Cauliflower (Flusher)

Celery

Collard greens (Anti-Bloater)

Cucumbers (Anti-Bloater)

Eggplant

Fennel

Green beans

Green peas

Greens: beet, collard, mustard, turnip (Anti-Bloater)

Kale (Anti-Bloater)

Leeks

Mushrooms

Mustard greens (Flusher, Anti-Bloater)

Onions

Parsley (Anti-Bloater)

Pumpkin (Flusher)

Romaine lettuce

Spinach (Flusher, Anti-Bloater)

Squash, spaghetti (Flusher)

Squash, yellow

String beans

Swiss chard

Tomatoes (Anti-Bloater, See list of tomato sauces [page 242] that qualify as Anti-Bloaters)

Turnip greens (Flusher, Anti-Bloater)

Zucchini

Fruit Flushers and Anti-Bloaters

Apples (Flusher)

Apricots (Anti-Bloater)

Bananas (Anti-Bloater)

Blackberries (Flusher)

Blueberries (Flusher)

Boysenberries (Flusher)

Cantaloupe (Anti-Bloater)

Cranberries (Anti-Bloater)

Currants (Flusher)

Elderberries (Flusher)

Figs (Flusher)

Gooseberries

Grapefruit (Anti-Bloater)

Grapes

Honeydew (Anti-Bloater)

Kiwifruit (Flusher, Anti-Bloater)

Lemons/Limes (Anti-Bloater)

Loganberries (Flusher)

Mango (Anti-Bloater)

Nectarines (Anti-Bloater)

Oranges (Flusher, Anti-Bloater)

Papaya (Anti-Bloater)

Pears (Flusher, Anti-Bloater)

Peaches (Anti-Bloater)

Pineapple

Plums (Anti-Bloater)

Plums, dried (prunes) (Flusher)

Raisins (Flusher, Anti-Bloater)

Raspberries (Flusher)

Strawberries (Flusher)

Watermelon (Anti-Bloater)

TOMATO SAUCES ("LOW-SODIUM" OR "NO SALT ADDED")

"Low-sodium" or "no salt added" tomato sauces or those with less than 140 milligrams and fewer than 50 calories per ½ cup are considered "non-starchy" and count as 1 Anti-Bloater or Flusher serving. (Those with 50 to 100 calories per ½ cup are similar to starchy vegetables and are counted as Carbohydrate Slimmers. See page 233.)

The Nitty-Gritty of Beverage Slimmers

	Your Weight (Pounds)	Servings per Day (approximate) (Men and Women)
Beverage Slimmers (Water or Tea)	125 pounds or less	8 (64 ounces)
	126–150	9 (72 ounces)
	151–175	10 (80 ounces)
	176–200	12 (98 ounces)
	201–225	14 (112 ounces)
	226–250	15 (120 ounces)
	251–300+	18 (144 ounces)

You need half of your body weight in fluid ounces daily. If you're 150 pounds, this means you need 75 fluid ounces a day, which is just over 9 cups. (There are 8 ounces in a cup.) *The good news?* This can come from both tea and water. Although you'll be getting fluid from your food, too, be sure to drink the recommended amount; our clients who meet these guidelines have had extraordinary health and weight-loss benefits. They also report feeling much more energetic and less hungry. Drinking 2 cups (16 ounces; many household glasses hold this much) of Beverage Slimmers at every meal, 2 cups with a snack or between meals, and 1 cup after dinner will give you 9 servings. (If you weigh more than 150 pounds, you'll need to fit a few more servings in throughout the day.) Five of your daily Beverage Slimmers servings should be green tea.

How do you know if you're properly hydrated? Your urine should be very light yellow, practically clear.

WATER

Your kidneys filter all of the vitamins, minerals, and nutrients that you eat. They work very hard all day, and because of this, the kidneys become less efficient with age. Think of your kidneys as a coffee filter: water can easily pass through. Imagine what happens when you dump salt on the filter. Very little salt, if any, will get through the filter on its own. Water is critical—when you pour water on the salt, the salt passes through the filter, cleansing it. Skimp on water and not only will your kidneys be overloaded, but the salt will back up in your tissues, creating major bloat and disease. Easy fix? Drink water to flush the salt.

If you drink tap water, the Environmental Protection Agency (EPA) has a draft guideline for sodium in drinking water of 20 milligrams per liter (mg/L). To find out how much sodium is in your public water supply, refer to the most recent Consumer Confidence Report, or contact your water supplier. Don't waste your money on bottled water since many pricey options are simply bottled tap water or not much better. If you're drinking sparkling water, be careful to check the labels as they contain sodium; choose those that have less than 10 milligrams of sodium per serving. If you use water softeners in your water, keep in mind that they do add sodium to your water; the harder the water, the more softener needed and the more sodium added. If you have very hard water you may want to consider only softening hot water and using unsoftened cold water for drinking and cooking. If you are looking to reduce impurities in your water, you can try a Brita filter.

TEA

Tea (green, black, and oolong) is unique—it's a calorie-free beverage and loaded with disease-fighting antioxidants called *flavonoids*. Herbal teas count as a Beverage Slimmer since they're calorie-free and sodium-free. However, herbal tea isn't really "tea." Unlike green, black, and oolong teas which all are made from the leaves of the tea bush, *Camellia sinensis,* herbal tea is actually an herbal infusion made from herbs and leaves other than the *Camellia senensis*. Green, black, and oolong teas are preferable since they contain the tea leaf, which offers a much higher antioxidant content and much more disease-fighting and metabolism-boosting potential.

Want healthy skin? Research shows that people who drink green tea regularly have less sun-related skin damage than those who don't. Brew a pitcher of iced tea and keep it refrigerated, so you'll always have refreshing tea ready.

Flavonoids fight cancer, heart disease, aging, inflammation, and the battle of the bulge. Tea plays an important role in increasing beneficial intestinal microflora (your body's "good" bacteria) as well as providing immunity against intestinal disorders and keeping your stomach distress- and bloat-free. Plus, if you drink *green* tea throughout the day, its powerful antioxidant, epigallocatechin gallate (EGCG), will rev your metabolism. It will take about 5 cups a day, but we know you can do it—at least during this Jumpstart phase. If you can't drink green tea, choose oolong or black tea or water, but realize that it is the green tea that really can rev your metabolism. Tea also makes your arteries more pliable, allowing blood and nutrients to travel more easily throughout your body, which in turn combats disease and rejuvenates cells (fights aging!) while de-bloating you.

Avoid adding sugar to your tea. The calories will add up too quickly when you're drinking 5 cups of tea or more a day. If you want to add a non-caloric sweetener like stevia, Equal, or Splenda, limit it to two packs a day.

Green tea has been used for centuries in China as a natural diuretic, and studies show green and oolong tea can lower your blood pressure and black tea can protect the health of your arteries. Also, all three teas contain the amino acid theanine, which helps to relax you and keep you alert, so it's the perfect morning brew. You'll be invigorated as you calmly start your day! Note: If for some reason you don't like tea, it's okay to drink water for all your Beverage Slimmer servings.

And if you opt for decaffeinated versions, that's okay, but realize that some of the studies reflecting green tea's metabolism-revving effects were seen with green tea's EGCG and caffeine combined.

Nutrition Twins FAVORITE

Lipton's Pyramid Green Tea with Mandarin Oranges and Lipton's Green Tea with Honey

COFFEE

We haven't forgotten about you coffee lovers. There's good news for you! You can have up to 12 ounces of coffee a day on the Jumpstart Plan. For some, the caffeine withdrawal would make this plan too difficult otherwise. You'll still lose the gut and the butt with your 12-ounce cup of Joe if you drink it black or add only skim milk (or a touch of fat-free creamer). Be sure to count that milk toward your Protein Slimmers servings. If you do drink coffee during the Jumpstart phase, remember that it is in *addition* to your Beverage Slimmer servings; you still need those 8+ servings of water or tea. Limit sugar to a maximum of one packet in your coffee per day. Better still, nix it. If you use artificial sweeteners, limit them to two packets a day. Cream, half-and-half, whole milk, and 2% milk are out, as are coffees with syrups.

The Nitty-Gritty of Freebies

During the Jumpstart phase, there are several foods that we consider "Freebies." If a food has less than 10 calories and less than 20 milligrams of sodium per serving, it's a Freebie. You can have up to 4 servings per day of any Freebie. Such foods include cooking spray, sugar-free jelly, sugar-free Jell-O, some nonfat dressings, and dressing sprays.

If you want a food that doesn't meet the requirements above and it contains 20 to 25 calories per serving and 40 milligrams or less of sodium (such as sugar-free syrup, light syrup, or some nonfat salad dressings), simply count 1 serving as two of your four daily Freebies.

Foods that you don't have to count and that you can have in unlimited quantities include spices with no added sodium, vinegars, and lemon juice. The best way to flavor your food is with spices. In fact, spices are so good for you that you can have as many as you'd like. Just don't use any type of salt (like sea salt or garlic salt), which is loaded with sodium! Not only are spices calorie free, fat free, and sodium free, they contain disease-fighting phytochemicals. So, not only do they make your food taste great, but they're good for you, too.

Spice It Up with These Low-Sodium Seasoning Blends

Try these seasoning blends at home to get delicious flavors without any fat, calories, or salt! For each seasoning blend, mix all ingredients and store in an airtight container. The ingredients call for dried herbs and ground spices unless otherwise noted. Each blend contains 5 milligrams of sodium or less per teaspoon.

Salt Shaker Blend #1
Makes 2½ tablespoons
1 tablespoon onion powder
1½ teaspoons basil
1½ teaspoons dry mustard
½ teaspoon chili powder
½ teaspoon ground celery seed
½ teaspoon paprika

Salt Shaker Blend #2
Makes 3 tablespoons
2 teaspoons thyme
2 teaspoons basil
2 teaspoons savory
1 tablespoon marjoram
1 teaspoon sage

Mediterranean Blend
Makes 4 teaspoons
½ teaspoon garlic powder
¼ teaspoon cayenne
½ teaspoon onion powder
1 teaspoon oregano
½ teaspoon cumin
½ teaspoon thyme
1 teaspoon coriander

Cooking Blend
Makes 2½ tablespoons
2 teaspoons thyme
1 teaspoon rosemary
1 tablespoon oregano
2 teaspoons dried minced onion
*Use 1 teaspoon for each pound of lean
    protein. Add ½ teaspoon for each
    2 quarts of soup.*

(continued)

(continued from previous page)

All-Purpose Blend
Makes 3 tablespoons
1 teaspoon celery seed
1 tablespoon basil
1 tablespoon marjoram
1 teaspoon onion powder
1 teaspoon thyme
Use 1 teaspoon per pound of protein.
   Use ½ teaspoon for 2 cups of
   vegetables.

Salad Blend
Makes 3⅓ tablespoons
1 tablespoon marjoram
1 teaspoon tarragon
2 teaspoons basil
1 teaspoon dill weed
1 tablespoon parsley
Sprinkle over tossed salads or add
   2 teaspoons for each cup of
   homemade salad dressing.

Adapted from www.RD411.com

Ready, Set, It's Drop Weight Time

By focusing on the Green Light foods in this chapter, you're soon going to feel slimmer, more energetic, younger, and happier. If you need more guidance or want to eliminate any planning, then follow the ten days of Jumpstart menus in the next chapter. When you're finished, you're going to feel fabulous.

Chapter 3

Ten Days of Jumpstart Plan Menus

You'll stay on the Jumpstart Plan for ten days and then move on to phase 2, the Maintenance Plan, which adds more calories and daily indulgences. The Jumpstart menus that follow provide 1,200 calories per day for women. Men will follow the same menus but will add more food, which is listed at the end of each daily menu. If you feel too hungry on the plan, you can add one Carbohydrate Slimmer or Protein Slimmer. Better yet, have an extra serving of vegetables. This works like a charm. Another way to keep your cravings in check is to have a bowl of our Anti-Bloat Broth (see recipe on page 221). It's salt free and very low in calories, and the veggies boost your nutrients.

Jumpstart Day 1 for Women

Breakfast

Warm peaches on cottage cheese and whole wheat bread:

⅓ cup warmed canned or fresh peaches *(canned in water or own juice, not syrup)*
(¾ Flusher/Anti-Bloater)

½ cup Friendship brand 1% milk fat cottage cheese (1 Protein Slimmer)

1 slice low-sodium whole wheat bread like Alvarado Street Bakery No Salt!
Sprouted Multi-Grain Bread (1 Carb Slimmer)

2 cups green tea or water (2 Beverage Slimmers)

Mid-Morning Snack

3 Ry-Krisp crackers (1 Carb Slimmer)

1 ounce *(3 slices)* extra thinly sliced, oven-roasted, low-sodium deli turkey breast
(such as Jennie-O Low-Sodium Turkey Breast) (½ Protein Slimmer)

2 cups green tea or water (2 Beverage Slimmers)

Lunch

Portabella mushroom burger made with:

1 large portabella mushroom cap (1 Flusher/Anti-Bloater)

Olive oil cooking spray (1 Freebie)

¾ ounce slice nonfat mozzarella cheese (¾ Protein Slimmer)

½ whole-grain bun *(bottom or top half)* (½ Carb Slimmer)

3 slices tomato (⅓ Flusher/Anti-Bloater)

3 leaves romaine lettuce (⅓ Flusher/Anti-Bloater)

3 slices onion (⅓ Flusher/Anti-Bloater)

To Make: Spray mushroom cap with olive oil cooking spray. Sauté mushroom cap
in nonstick skillet with olive oil cooking spray. Cook on medium heat until juices
start to drip from the mushroom caps, about 5 minutes. Turn caps over and continue to cook until mushrooms are flexible and no longer firm when pressed, 5 to
7 minutes longer. Top with cheese slice and allow cheese to melt. Remove from
heat and place on ½ of whole-grain bun. Top with tomato, lettuce, and onion.

Strawberry Salad made with:

1 cup chopped romaine lettuce (1 Flusher/Anti-Bloater)

½ cup sliced strawberries (1 Flusher/Anti-Bloater)

1 teaspoon olive oil ($\frac{1}{3}$ Mono Slimmer)

Balsamic vinegar to taste (Unlimited Freebie)

1 tablespoon slivered almonds ($\frac{1}{2}$ Mono Slimmer)

1 cup green tea, 1 cup water (2 Beverage Slimmers)

Mid-Afternoon Snack

3 cups air-popped popcorn, no butter or oil added (1 Carb Slimmer)

I Can't Believe It's Not Butter! spray, misted lightly on popcorn (Freebie)

1 large bell pepper, cut in strips (1 Flusher/Anti-Bloater)

2 cups green tea (2 Beverage Slimmers)

Dinner

Salmon with dill, steamed spinach, mashed red potatoes made with:

¼ cup plain nonfat yogurt ($\frac{1}{3}$ Protein Slimmer)

¼ teaspoon dill, dried (Unlimited)

½ teaspoon lemon juice (Unlimited)

¼ teaspoon Mrs. Dash Original or Lemon and Pepper (Unlimited)

3 ounces salmon fillet (2 Protein Slimmers)

1 cup Nutrition Twins Skinny Mashed Potatoes *(see recipe page 218)* (1 Carb Slimmer)

1 cup steamed spinach (2 Flushers/Anti-Bloaters)

1 cup water (1 Beverage Slimmer)

2 cups green tea (2 Beverage Slimmers)

To Make: Preheat oven to 350° F. Whisk together yogurt, dill, lemon juice, and Mrs. Dash. Pour over salmon fillet. Bake 15 to 18 minutes until done. You can test for readiness by checking it with a fork; when it's done it will be uniformly opaque in the thickest part of the fish and it will flake easily. Serve over steamed spinach, spritzed with lemon, if desired, along with mashed potatoes.

After-Dinner Snack *(at least an hour before bed)* •••••••••••••••••••••••••••••••••••

½ cup cubed cantaloupe (½ Flusher/Anti-Bloater)

6 ounces Stonyfield Farm plain nonfat yogurt (1 Protein Slimmer)

1 cup green tea (1 Beverage Slimmer)

> DAILY TOTAL: Calories 1,172, Carbohydrates 165 grams, Protein 87 grams, Fat 22 grams,
> Saturated Fat 5 grams, Fiber 26 grams, Sodium 1,250 milligrams
> 4 Carb Slimmers, 5¼ Protein Slimmers, ⅚ Mono Slimmers, 8 Flushers/Anti-Bloaters,
> 9 Beverage Slimmers, 2 Freebies

Jumpstart Day 1 Men

Breakfast: Have two slices of bread instead of one. **Mid-morning snack:** Add
an extra ounce of low-sodium turkey. **Dinner:** Add 1½ extra ounces of
salmon and an extra ¾ cup steamed spinach.

> DAILY TOTAL: Calories 1,400, Carbohydrates 190 grams, Protein 115 grams, Fat 26 grams,
> Saturated Fat 6 grams, Fiber 35 grams, Sodium 1,498 milligrams
> 5 Carb Slimmers, 6¾ Protein Slimmers, ⅚ Mono Slimmer, 9½ Flushers/Anti-Bloaters,
> 9 Beverage Slimmers, 2 Freebies

Jumpstart Day 2 Women

Breakfast ••

¾ cup Kashi Go Lean (1 Carb Slimmer)

1 cup skim milk (1 Protein Slimmer)

¼ cup blueberries (½ Flusher/Anti-Bloater)

2 cups green tea (2 Beverage Slimmers)

Lunch ••

"Grilled" Cheese and Veggie-Apple Pita Sandwich, with celery and carrot sticks:
1 Trader Joes' 100% Whole Wheat Apocryphal Pita (1½ Carb Slimmers)
1 ounce Polly-O Nonfat Mozzarella Cheese (1 Protein Slimmer)

¾ cup shredded romaine lettuce (³/₄ Flusher/Anti-Bloater)

¼ cup shredded carrots (¼ Flusher/Anti-Bloater)

½ apple diced (½ Flusher/Anti-Bloater)

20 squirts Wishbone Salad Italian Vinaigrette Spray (Freebie)

1 cup celery and carrot sticks (1 Flusher/Anti-Bloater)

1 cup water, 1 cup green tea (2 Beverage Slimmers)

To Make: Cut pita bread in half and fill each pocket with cheese. Turn toaster oven to medium-high and bake pita and cheese until cheese melts. Take pita out of toaster and add lettuce, carrots, and apple; spray dressing in each pocket. Serve with celery and carrots.

Mid-Afternoon Snack

1 Ryvita Rye and Oatbran Crispbread (½ Carb Slimmer)

¼ cup Friendship Low-Fat, Low-Sodium Cottage Cheese mixed with chives
   (½ Protein Slimmer)

1 cup water (1 Beverage Slimmer)

Dinner

Baja Fish Tacos with Mango Salsa *(see recipe page 181)* (1 Carb Slimmer,
   2 Protein Slimmers, 1 Flusher/Anti-Bloater)

1½ cups steamed zucchini, yellow squash, and red bell pepper with crushed
   garlic and cilantro (3 Flushers/Anti-Bloaters)

1 cup water, 1 cup green tea (2 Beverage Slimmers)

After-Dinner Snack *(at least an hour before bed)*

6 ounces Dannon Light and Fit Yogurt, Vanilla (1 Protein Slimmer)

2 tablespoons slivered almonds (1 Mono Slimmer)

DAILY TOTAL: Calories 1,152, Fat 25 grams, Carbohydrates 163 grams, Protein 92 grams,
Saturated Fat 4 grams, Fiber 34.5 grams, Sodium 1,210 milligrams
4 Carb Slimmers, 5½ Protein Slimmers, 1 Mono Slimmer, 7 Flushers/Anti-Bloaters,
9 Beverage Slimmers, 1 Freebie

Jumpstart Day 2 Men

Breakfast: Add an additional ¾ cup Kashi Go Lean and ½ cup milk. **Lunch:**
Add a hard-boiled egg to your veggie and apple pita.

DAILY TOTAL: Calories 1,383, Carbohydrates 192 grams, Protein 113 grams, Fat 31 grams,
Saturated Fat 6 grams, Fiber 42.3 grams, Sodium 1,401.1 milligrams
5 Carb Slimmers, 7 Protein Slimmers, 1 Mono Slimmer, 7 Flushers/Anti-Bloaters, 9 Beverage
Slimmers, 1 Freebie

Jumpstart Day 3 Women

Breakfast

4 Blueberry Protein Pancakes *(see recipe page 204)* (1½ Carb Slimmers, 1½ Protein
   Slimmers, 1 Flusher/Anti-Bloater)

2 tablespoons sugar-free syrup *(optional)* (Freebie)

2 cups green tea (2 Beverage Slimmers)

Lunch

Citrus Chicken and Walnut Salad made with:

2 cups spinach (2 Flushers/Anti-Bloaters)

½ cup each sliced bell peppers, broccoli, tomato, and cucumber
   (2 Flushers/Anti-Bloaters)

2 ounces chicken breast, cut into strips (1 Protein Slimmer)

1 orange, cut into pieces (1 Flusher/Anti-Bloater)

1 tablespoon slivered walnuts (½ Mono Slimmer)

1 teaspoon olive oil, sprayed onto salad (⅓ Mono Slimmer)

To Make: Toss all ingredients together.

6 Health Valley rice bran graham crackers (1 Carb Slimmer)

2 cups green tea (2 Beverage Slimmers)

Mid-Afternoon Snack

5 cups popped Smart Balance Smart 'n Healthy microwave popcorn
(1 Carb Slimmer)

1 cup green tea, 1 cup water (2 Beverage Slimmers)

Dinner

1 cup Ore Ida Steam 'n Mash Cut Sweet Potato (1 Carb Slimmer)

1 serving Grilled Lemon Pepper Herb Salmon *(See recipe page 186)*
(2 Protein Slimmers)

1 cup steamed broccoli and carrots (2 Flushers/Anti-Bloaters) with basil

2 cups water (2 Beverage Slimmers)

After-Dinner Snack *(at least an hour before bed)*

2 Peaches and Cream Pops *(See recipe page 201)* (2 pops = ½ Flusher/Anti-Bloater,
½ Protein Slimmer)

1 water (1 Beverage Slimmer)

DAILY TOTAL: Calories 1,194, Carbohydrates 179 grams, Protein 85 grams, Total Fat 25 grams, Saturated Fat 3 grams, Fiber 33 grams, Sodium 1,066 milligrams
4 Carb Slimmers, 4¾ Protein Slimmers, 8½ Flushers/Anti-Bloaters. ⅙ Mono Slimmer, 9 Beverage Slimmers, 1 Freebie

Jumpstart Day 3 Men

Lunch: Add an extra ounce of chicken to your salad and have an extra 6 Health Valley Rice Bran Graham Crackers. **Dinner:** Have an additional two ounces of salmon.

DAILY TOTAL: Calories 1,431, Carbohydrates 198 grams, Protein 109 grams, Total Fat 33 grams, Saturated Fat 3 grams, Fiber 36 grams, Sodium 1,236 milligrams
5 Carb Slimmers, 6¼ Protein Slimmers, 8½ Flushers/Anti-Bloaters, 1 Mono Slimmer, 9 Beverage Slimmers, 1 Freebie

Jumpstart Day 4 Women

Breakfast •••

1 packet Quaker Instant Organic Oatmeal (1 Carb Slimmer)

Scrambled egg white and veggie omelet made with:

4 egg whites (1 Protein Slimmer)

¾ cup spinach and sliced mushrooms (¾ Flusher)

Cooking spray *(for pan)*

½ apple (½ Flusher/Anti-Bloater)

1 cup green tea, 1 cup water (2 Beverage Slimmers)

Lunch •••

Pita Pizza made with:

Trader Joe's Organic 100% Whole Wheat Pita *(open it to have two flat pieces)*
    (1 Carb Slimmer)

½ cup Walnut Acres Low Sodium Tomato and Basil Pasta Sauce
    (1 Anti-Bloater/Flusher)

1½ ounces low-fat Swiss cheese (1½ Protein Slimmers)

½ cup sliced mushrooms and bell peppers for pizza topping (½ Flusher/Anti-Bloater)

½ cup spinach for pizza topping (½ Flusher/Anti-Bloater)

½ banana (1 Flusher/Anti-Bloater)

1 cup sliced cucumber and cherry tomatoes (1 Flusher/Anti-Bloater)

1 cup water, 1 cup green tea (2 Beverage Slimmers)

Snack •••

1 Ryvita dark Rye Crispbread (½ Carb Slimmer)

½ ounce farmers cheese (½ Protein Slimmer)

2 cups green tea (2 Beverage Slimmers)

Dinner ••

Mediterranean Salmon made with:

3 ounces baked salmon (2 Protein Slimmers)

Sprinkle Mediterranean Blend Spices (optional) *(see recipe on page 45)*

To Make: Preheat oven to Broil. Spray a shallow-sided aluminum baking pan with olive oil spray and the top of the salmon. Broil (on the top rack) for about 10–15 minutes, without turning, until the edges of the fish are browned, the flesh is a whitish pink (no longer clear), and it flakes when touched with a fork.

¼ cup brown rice, cooked (½ Carb Slimmer)

1 cup tomato and cucumber salad, seasoned with vinegar and lemon
   (1 Flusher/Anti-Bloater)

1 cup steamed asparagus and string beans with dill weed (2 Flushers/Anti-Bloaters)

1 ear corn on the cob (1 Carb Slimmer)

2 cups water (2 Beverage Slimmers)

After-Dinner Snack *(at least an hour before bed)*

1 baked D'anjou pear with cinnamon (1 Flusher/Anti-Bloater)

2 tablespoons slivered almonds (1 Mono Slimmer)

1 cup green tea (1 Beverage Slimmer)

> DAILY TOTAL: Calories 1,189, Total Carbohydrates 174 grams, Protein 78 grams, Total Fat 28 grams, Saturated Fat 5.5 grams, Fiber 38 grams, Sodium 1,083 milligrams
> 4 Carb Slimmers, 5 Protein Slimmers, 1 Mono Slimmer, 7¾ Flushers/Anti-Bloaters,
> 9 Beverage Slimmers

Jumpstart Day 4 Men

Snack: Have two Ryvita Crispbread rather than one. **Dinner:** Have an extra 2¼ ounces of salmon and an extra ¼ cup brown rice.

> DAILY TOTAL: Calories 1,405, Total Carbohydrates 194 grams, Protein 98 grams, Total Fat 34 grams, Saturated Fat 6 grams, Fiber 42 grams, Sodium 1,500 milligrams
> 5 Carb Slimmers, 6½ Protein Slimmers, 1 Mono Slimmer, 7¾ Flushers/Anti-Bloaters,
> 9 Beverage Slimmers

Jumpstart Day 5 Women

Breakfast

Farmer's Market Omelet *(See recipe page 206)* (1 serving equals ½ of the recipe)
(2 Protein Slimmers, 1 Flusher/Anti-Bloater)

1 slice Pepperidge Farm Stoneground 100% Whole Wheat Small Slice Bread
(1 Carb Slimmer)

2 cups green tea (2 Beverage Slimmers)

Lunch

⅔ cup Chicken Salad *(See recipe page 209)* (1 Protein Slimmer)

1 small Trader Joe's Organic 100% Whole Wheat Pita (1 Carb Slimmer)

Lemon wedge to squeeze in sandwich (Unlimited)

1 cup grape tomatoes and bell peppers, cut into strips (1 Flusher/Anti-Bloater)

½ cup baby carrots (½ Flusher/Anti-Bloater)

1 peach (1 Flusher/Anti-Bloater)

1 cup of green tea and 1 cup water (2 Beverage Slimmers)

Mid-Afternoon Snack

6-ounce container 0% Fage Greek Yogurt (1 Protein Slimmer)

¼ cup sliced strawberries (½ Flusher/Anti-Bloater)

2 cups green tea (2 Beverage Slimmers)

Dinner

Almond-Crusted Shrimp *(See recipe page 178)* (½ Carb Slimmer, 1½ Protein Slimmers, 1 Mono Slimmer)

¾ cup brown rice (½ Carb Slimmer)

1 cup grilled asparagus (1 Flusher/Anti-Bloater)

1 cup grilled sliced eggplant *(spray cooking spray on asparagus and eggplant; grill or roast)* (1 Flusher/Anti-Bloater)

2 cups green tea (2 Beverage Slimmers)

After-Dinner Snack *(at least an hour before bed)* •

1 Peaches and Cream Pop *(See recipe page 201)* (1 pop = ¼ Flusher/Anti-Bloater)

1 water (1 Beverage Slimmer)

> DAILY TOTAL: Calories 1,205, Carbohydrates 145 grams, Protein 79 grams, Total Fat 36 grams, Saturated Fat 6 grams, Fiber 28 grams, Sodium 870 milligrams
> 4 Carb Slimmers, 5½ Protein Slimmers, 1 Mono Slimmer, 6½ Flushers/Anti-Bloaters, 9 Beverage Slimmers

Jumpstart Day 5 Men

Lunch: Have an additional ¼ cup of chicken salad. **Afternoon snack:** Have an additional ¼ cup sliced berries (count as ½ Carb Slimmer). **Dinner:** Have 1½ servings of the shrimp recipe rather than 1 serving. (Count the extra ½ Mono Slimmer from the recipe as ½ Protein Slimmer.)

> DAILY TOTAL: Calories 1,410, Carbohydrates 155 grams, Protein 94 grams, Fat 44 grams, Saturated Fat 7 grams, Fiber 33 grams, Sodium 942 milligrams
> 4¾ Carb Slimmers, 6½ Protein Slimmer (½ Mono Slimmers count towards Protein), 1½ Mono Slimmers, 7½ Flushers/Anti-Bloaters, 9 Beverage Slimmers

Jumpstart Day 6 Women

Breakfast •

Yogurt Crunch made by stirring cereal into yogurt:

1 5.8-ounce container 0% Fage Greek Yogurt (1 Protein Slimmer)

⅔ cup Nature's Path Organic Synergy 8 Whole Grains (1 Carb Slimmer)

1 small banana (1 Flusher/Anti-Bloater)

2 cups water (2 Beverage Slimmers)

Lunch •

Rice, tomato, and bean salad made with:

¾ cup cooked brown rice (1½ Carb Slimmers)

1 teaspoon canola oil (⅓ Mono Slimmer)

2 cloves garlic, sautéed (¼ Flusher/Anti-Bloater)

2 tomatoes, diced and sautéed (1 Flusher/Anti-Bloater)

½ cup cooked northern white beans, rinsed and drained (1 Protein Slimmer)

1 tablespoon low-sodium salsa like Frog Ranch Low Sodium Salsa, optional

To Make: Sauté the garlic and tomatoes in canola oil, then stir in beans and pour the mixture over the rice. Serve with salsa, if desired.

1½ cups raw zucchini and carrot sticks (1½ Flushers/Anti-Bloaters)

2 cups green tea and 1 cup water (3 Beverage Slimmers)

Mid-Afternoon Snack

Peachy Shake made with:

6 ounces nonfat light yogurt, peach flavor (1 Protein Slimmer)

1 peach, sliced and frozen *(or 1 cup frozen sliced peaches)* (1 Flusher/Anti-Bloater)

To Make: Blend yogurt and fruit with a few pieces of ice to make a shake.

1 cup green tea (1 Beverage Slimmer)

Dinner

2 cups mixed greens with lemon and balsamic vinegar
(2 Flushers/Anti-Bloaters, Freebies)

One serving of Avocado and Grapefruit Chicken *(See recipe page 180)*
(1½ Protein Slimmers, 1½ Carb Slimmers, ½ Mono Slimmer, ½ Flusher/Anti-Bloater)

1 cup of green tea, 1 cup of water (2 Beverage Slimmers)

After-Dinner Snack *(at least an hour before bed)*

10 unsalted pistachios (⅓ Mono Slimmer)

½ Sargento Light String cheese (½ Protein Slimmer)

1 cup of green tea (1 Beverage Slimmer)

DAILY TOTAL: Calories 1,203, Carbohydrates 207 grams, Protein 62 grams, Fat 20 grams, Saturated Fat 3 grams, Fiber 30 grams, Sodium 728 milligrams
4 Carb Slimmers, 5 Protein Slimmers, 1⅓ Mono Slimmers, 7¼ Flushers/Anti-Bloaters, 9 Beverage Slimmers

Jumpstart Day 6 Men

Lunch: Add ½ cup white northern beans. **Mid-afternoon snack:** Add 1 cup strawberries to the shake. **After-dinner snack:** Add ½ Sargento Light String cheese.

DAILY TOTAL: Calories 1,401, Carbohydrates 241 grams, Protein 75 grams, Fat 22 grams, Saturated Fat 4 grams, Fiber 38 grams, Sodium 980 milligrams
5 Carb Slimmers, 6½ Protein Slimmers, 1⅓ Mono Slimmers, 8¼ Flushers/Anti-Bloaters, 9 Beverage Slimmers

Jumpstart Day 7 Women

Breakfast

Quaker Instant plain oatmeal sprinkled with cinnamon (1 Carb Slimmer)

1 5.3-ounce 0% Fage Greek Yogurt (1 Protein Slimmer)

1 small grapefruit (1 Flusher/Anti-Bloater)

1 cup green tea and 1 cup water (2 Beverage Slimmers)

Lunch

Spinach and Mango Salad made with:

2 cups fresh spinach (2 Flushers/Anti-Bloaters)

½ large mango, cut in slices (1 Flusher/Anti-Bloater)

1 teaspoon olive oil (⅓ Mono Slimmer)

Splash balsamic vinegar (Unlimited)

Squirt lemon (Unlimited)

The Nutrition Twins Skinny Rice Pilaf
   (See recipe page 219) (1 Carb Slimmers, ⅓ Mono Slimmer) **topped with:**

1½ ounces grilled pork tenderloin (1 Protein Slimmer)

1 cup steamed string beans, mushrooms, and sugar snap peas
   (2 Flushers/Anti-Bloaters)

1 cup water, 1 cup green tea (2 Beverage Slimmers)

Mid-Afternoon Snack ··

Hummus and turkey lettuce wrap made with:

1 tablespoon hummus (⅓ Mono Slimmer)

2 ounces Boar's Head 47% Less Sodium Turkey Breast (1 Protein Slimmer)

1 lettuce leaf (¼ Flusher/Anti-Bloater)

2 cups of water (2 Beverage Slimmers)

Dinner ··

Pasta and meat sauce with vegetables made with:

½ cup whole wheat pasta *(cooked)* (1 Carb Slimmer)

1 cup steamed broccoli florets (2 Flushers/Anti-Bloaters)

¼ cup steamed mushrooms (½ Flusher/Anti-Bloater)

¼ cup steamed spinach (½ Flusher/Anti-Bloater)

3 ounces ground round, extra lean (2 Protein Slimmers)

1 cup Del Monte Tomato Sauce No Salt Added, seasoned with garlic powder, oregano, and black pepper to taste (2 Flushers/Anti-Bloaters)

1 cup steamed carrots and broccoli (2 Flushers/Anti-Bloaters)

1 cup green tea, 1 cup water (2 Beverage Slimmers)

After-Dinner Snack *(at least an hour before bed)* ····················

3 Health Valley Rice Bran Graham Crackers, Original (½ Carb Slimmer)

1 teaspoon unsalted sunflower nut butter or peanut butter (⅓ Mono Slimmer)

1 cup green tea (1 Beverage Slimmer)

DAILY TOTAL: Calories 1,250, Carbohydrates 165 grams, Protein 90 grams, Fat 32 grams, Saturated Fat 6 grams, Fiber 34 grams, Sodium 880 milligrams
3½ Carb Slimmers, 5 Protein Slimmers, 1⅓ Mono Slimmers, 11¼ Flushers/Anti-Bloaters, 9 Beverage Slimmers

Jumpstart Day 7 Men

Breakfast: Add another packet of Quaker's plain instant oatmeal. **Lunch:** Add another 1½ ounces of pork tenderloin. **Dinner:** Add another ¾ ounce of ground round.

> DAILY TOTAL: Calories 1,449, Carbohydrates 184 grams, Protein 111 grams, Fat 37 grams, Saturated Fat 7 grams, Fiber 37 grams, Sodium 995 milligrams
> 4½ Carb Slimmers, 6½ Protein Slimmers, 1⅓ Mono Slimmers, 11¼ Flushers/Anti-Bloaters, 9 Beverage Slimmers

Jumpstart Day 8 Women

Breakfast

The Nutrition Twins Skinny Peanut Butter Banana Roll-Up *(See recipe page 200)*
(1 Carb Slimmer, 1 Mono Slimmer, 1 Flusher/Anti-Bloater)

2 cups water, 1 cup green tea (3 Beverage Slimmers)

Mid-Morning Snack

15 pods edamame beans (½ Protein Slimmer)

1 cup carrot and celery sticks (1 Flusher/Anti-Bloater)

1 cup green tea (1 Beverage Slimmer)

Lunch

Melted cheese sandwich made with:

2 slices Pepperidge Farm Stoneground 100% Whole Wheat bread *(2 Carb Slimmers)*

1 ounce Polly-O Fat-Free Mozzarella Cheese or low-fat Swiss cheese or Cabot's 75% Light Cheddar Cheese (1 Protein Slimmer)

Lettuce, tomato, and peppers on sandwich (¼ Flusher/Anti-Bloater)

1 orange (1 Flusher/Anti-Bloater)

1 cup steamed vegetable medley *(cauliflower, carrots, broccoli, and asparagus)*
(2 Flushers/Anti-Bloaters) seasoned with Mrs. Dash, lemon, and pepper
(Unlimited Freebies)

1 cup green tea, 1 cup water (2 Beverage Slimmers)

Mid-Afternoon Snack

6 ounces Dannon Light 'n Fit yogurt (1 Protein Slimmer)

1 cup zucchini and squash strips (1 Flusher/Anti-Bloater)

1 cup water (1 Beverage Slimmer)

Dinner

Dinner salad made with:

2 cups romaine lettuce (2 Flushers/Anti-Bloaters)

½ cup cherry tomatoes (½ Flusher/Anti-Bloater)

¼ cup chopped bell peppers (¼ Flusher/Anti-Bloater)

Lemon and balsamic vinegar to taste (Unlimited Freebies)

1 serving *(about 1 cup)* of The Nutrition Twins Skinny Rosemary Turkey with
   Vegetables *(see recipe on page 195)* (1¾ Protein Slimmers, 1 Flusher/Anti-Bloater)

1 serving of The Nutrition Twins Skinny Mashed Potatoes *(see recipe on
   page 218)* (1 Carb Slimmer)

1 cup water, 1 cup green tea (2 Beverage Slimmers)

After-Dinner Snack *(at least an hour before bed)*

4 ounces Oikos Organic Greek Style yogurt (¾ Protein Slimmer)

1 cup green tea (1 Beverage Slimmer)

DAILY TOTAL: Calories 1,184, Carbohydrates 182 grams, Protein 80 grams, Fat 23 grams,
Saturated Fat 5 grams, Fiber 28 grams, Sodium 844 milligrams
4 Carb Slimmers, 5 Protein Slimmers, 1 Mono Slimmer, 8¾ Flushers/Anti-Bloaters,
10 Beverage Slimmers

Jumpstart Day 8 Men

Mid-morning Snack: Add 15 extra edamame pods. **Lunch:** Add 1 ounce more
   cheese. **Dinner:** Add an extra serving *(approximately 1 cup)* of The Nutrition
   Twins Skinny Mashed Potatoes

DAILY TOTAL: Calories 1,410, Carbohydrates 212 grams, Protein 96 grams, Fat 28 grams,
Saturated Fat 6 grams, Fiber 33 grams, Sodium 953 milligrams
5 Carb Slimmers, 6½ Protein Slimmers, 1 Mono Slimmer, 8¾ Flushers/Anti-Bloaters,
10 Beverage Slimmers

Jumpstart Day 9 Women

Breakfast

½ cup Fiber One or ¾ Cup Heart to Heart mixed into: (1 Carb Slimmer)

1 5.8-ounce 0% Fage Greek Yogurt (1 Protein Slimmer)

½ cup sliced strawberries (1 Flusher/Anti-Bloater)

2 cups green tea (2 Beverage Slimmers)

Lunch

Turkey Hummus Wheel made with:

1 Tumaro's Gourmet Tortillas-Soy-Ful Heart Flatbread *(or other whole-grain tortilla with less than 100 calories and less than 110 mg sodium)* (1 Carb Slimmer)

2 ounces fresh sliced turkey breast (1 Protein Slimmer)

2 level tablespoons hummus (²/₃ Mono Slimmer)

½ cup chopped tomato (½ Flusher/Anti-Bloater)

½ cup chopped romaine lettuce (½ Flusher/Anti-Bloater)

Spread hummus on a tortilla. Add turkey, tomato, and lettuce and roll up.

Salad made with:

1 cup romaine lettuce (1 Flusher/Anti-Bloater)

½ cup each shredded carrot, squash, asparagus (1½ Flushers/Anti-Bloaters)

1 tablespoon Vinaigrette Salad Dressing *(see recipe page 224)* (1½ Freebies)

1 cup green tea, 1 cup water (2 Beverage Slimmers)

Mid-Afternoon Snack

4 Sunsweet Ones Dried Plums (1 Flusher/Anti-Bloater)

10 pistachios (⅓ Mono Slimmer)

2 cups green tea (2 Beverage Slimmers)

Dinner

1 serving The Nutrition Twins Skinny Chicken Parm *(See recipe page 193)*
(2 Protein Slimmers, ½ Carb Slimmer, 1 Flusher/Anti-Bloater)

1 slice Ezekiel 4:9 Organic Sprouted Whole Grain Sesame Bread *(or other whole-grain roll or bread with less than 100 calories and less than 110 mg sodium)*
(1 Carb Slimmer)

2 cups kale sautéed in 3 tablespoons Nutrition Twins Skinny Anti-Bloat Broth *(see recipe page 221)* (2 Flushers/Anti-Bloaters, ½ Freebie)

1 cup The Nutrition Twins Skinny Cauliflower Mash (2 Flushers/Anti-Bloaters)

2 cups water (2 Beverage Slimmers)

After-Dinner Snack *(at least an hour before bed)*

1 slice Ryvita Rye and Oat Bran Crispbread (½ Carb Slimmer)

1 The Laughing Cow, Mini Babybel, Light Original (1 Protein Slimmer)

1 cup green tea (1 Beverage Slimmer)

> DAILY TOTAL: Calories 1,234, Carbohydrates 181 grams, Protein 99 grams, Fat 26 grams, Saturated Fat 7 grams, Fiber 42 grams, Sodium 1,229 milligrams
> 4 Carb Slimmers, 5 Protein Slimmers, 10 Flushers/Anti-Bloaters, 1 Mono Slimmer, 9 Beverage Slimmers, 2 Freebies

Jumpstart Day 9 Men

Breakfast: Add an additional ⅓ cup Kashi Heart to Heart. **Lunch:** Add an extra 3 ounces of turkey.

> DAILY TOTAL: Calories 1,435, Carbohydrates 193 grams, Protein 129 grams, Fat 30 grams, Saturated Fat 8 grams, Fiber 44 grams, Sodium 1,288 milligrams
> 5 Carb Slimmers, 6½ Protein Slimmers, 10 Flushers/Anti-Bloaters, 1 Mono Slimmer, 9 Beverage Slimmers, 2 Freebies

Jumpstart Day 10 Women

Breakfast

Quick Muesli made with:

6 ounces non-fat plain yogurt (1 Protein Slimmer)

4 chopped almonds (⅓ Mono Slimmer)

1 orange, sectioned and sliced (1 Flusher/Anti-Bloater)

1 tablespoon raisins (⅓ Flusher/Anti-Bloater)

Dash Cinnamon

To Make: Mix all ingredients together and enjoy!

1 cup water, 2 cups green tea (3 Beverage Slimmers)

Lunch

3 ounces *(1 serving)* Creamy Sun-Dried Tomato Tuna Salad *(See recipe page 210)*
   (1½ Protein Slimmers, ½ Mono Slimmer, 1 Flusher/Anti-Bloater)

1 Trader Joe's Organic 100% Whole Wheat Pita (1 Carb Slimmer)

1½ cups steamed carrots, cauliflower, and broccoli (3 Flushers/Anti-Bloaters)

1 cup water, 1 cup green tea (2 Beverage Slimmers)

Snack

6 Health Valley Rice Bran Graham Crackers, Original (1 Carb Slimmer)

The Laughing Cow, Mini Babybel, Light Original, spread over crackers
   (1 Protein Slimmer)

1 cup green tea (1 Beverage Slimmer)

Dinner

1 serving Gold Coast Autumn Salad with California Figs *(See recipe page 211)*
   (1¼ Flushers/Anti-Bloaters)

3 ounces chicken breast, grilled or baked (1½ Protein Slimmers)

¾ cup wild rice (1½ Carb Slimmers)

1½ cups sautéed kale *(sauté in olive oil and Nutrition Twins Skinny Anti-Bloat Broth, see recipe page 221)* (3 Flushers/Anti-Bloaters)

½ teaspooon olive oil for sauteéing (⅙ Mono Slimmer)

1 cup green tea, 1 cup water (2 Beverage Slimmers)

After-Dinner Snack *(at least an hour before bed)* •••••••••••••••••••••••••••••••••••

1 cup of celery and carrots stalks (1 Flusher/Anti-Bloater)

1 cup green tea (1 Beverage Slimmer)

DAILY TOTAL: Calories 1,218, Carbohydrates 171 grams, Protein 74 grams, Fat 29 grams, Saturated Fat 6 grams, Fiber 30 grams, Sodium 885 milligrams
4⅓ Carb Slimmers, 5 Protein Slimmers, 1 Mono Slimmer, 10½ Flushers/Anti-Bloaters, 9 Beverage Slimmers

Jumpstart Day 10 Men

Have an additional 3 ounces chicken with dinner and an additional ½ cup wild rice.

DAILY TOTAL: Calories 1,426, Carbohydrates 188 grams, Protein 112 grams, Fat 31 grams, Saturated Fat 6 grams, Fiber 32 grams, Sodium 930 milligrams
5⅓ Carb Slimmers, 6½ Protein Slimmers, 1 Mono Slimmer, 10½ Anti-Bloaters/Flushers, 9 Beverage Slimmers

Chapter **4**

Becoming Salt-Savvy: Salt-Slashing and Sleuthing in the Real World

All tastes are acquired. We develop our taste preferences soon after birth, and they continue to develop depending on the foods we're exposed to. If you were frequently exposed to salty meals, there's a good chance that you acquired a taste for them. The good news is that our taste buds, like all other cells in the body, experience "turnover," which means they continuously die and are replaced. So if you go on a low-sodium diet for several weeks, your new taste buds will adjust for the better. In fact, it normally takes about 21 days for your taste buds to turn over, so it's quite likely that by the time you are finished with the Jumpstart phase of the plan, you will be on your way to decreased cravings for salty foods.

Surefire Salt Stand-Ins

- A celery stalk with 1 teaspoon of all-natural, unsalted peanut butter (*½ Flusher/Anti- Bloater, ⅓ Mono Slimmer*)
- 30 unsalted pistachios or other nuts sprinkled with the Saltshaker Blend #1 (*See recipe page 45*) (*1 Mono Slimmer*)
- 3 brown rice cakes sprinkled with cinnamon, paprika, cardamom, cayenne, and coriander (*1 Carb Slimmer*)
- 3 cups unsalted, air-popped popcorn seasoned with cayenne powder, onion powder, garlic powder, chili powder, coriander, and cumin, or sprinkled with chili powder and paprika (*1 Carb Slimmer*)
- 1 small (*3½-ounce*) baked potato with pepper or paprika (*1 Carb Slimmer*)

Curbing Your Cravings

So what do you do in the meantime when you crave a salty snack? Try the salt stand-ins on the left.

If you're more apt to crave sugar than salt, here's some good news: For every kind of candy you love, there's a fruit that can give you nearly the same taste sensation and mouth-feel that will totally satisfy you. Best of all, because fruit contains far less insulin-spiking sugar and is packed with fiber, you'll feel fuller longer! So, what's your candy craving?

If You Crave:	Eat This:
Chocolate	Fresh dates or figs rolled in cocoa powder (4 dates or 2 large figs (or 3 small figs) = 1 Flusher/ Anti-Bloater serving)
Tangy sweets, such as Starburst, Skittles, or Mike and Ike	Kiwi, pineapple, mango (2 kiwi, ¾ cup chopped pineapple, or ½ mango = 1 Flusher/ Anti-Bloater serving)
A tart candy, such as SweeTarts or Smarties	Grapefruit, tart dried cherries, or pomegranate (1 small grapefruit, ½ pomegranate, or ¼ cup unsweetened tart dried cherries = 1 Flusher/Anti-Bloater serving)
A soft and gooey sweet, such as marshmallows, jelly beans, or caramel	Fresh dates or dried apricots or dried plums (4 dates, 4 dried apricots, or 4 dried plums = 1 Flusher/Anti-Bloater serving)
Pure sugar, such as cotton candy	Sugar-packed fruits, such as an overripe frozen banana, or raisins (1 small banana or ¼ cup raisins = 1 Flusher/Anti-Bloater)

Becoming Salt-Savvy in the Real World

No matter where you are—at home, the supermarket, or dining out—there are things you can do to avoid foods that are very high in sodium. All it takes is a little awareness. Sodium occurs naturally in some foods and is added to many others. Nuts, grains, fruits, and vegetables all naturally contain low amounts of sodium, but you'll often find that these foods are high in sodium after they've been processed. Flavored rice mixes, seasoned meats and nuts, frozen vegetables with sauces, and canned vegetables and fruits are just a few examples of foods with high amounts of sodium listed on their Nutrition Facts label. Baking soda, soy sauce, garlic salt, and Worcestershire sauce are just a few examples of salt sources added to many of your favorite foods. But just because foods have sodium added to them doesn't mean they're necessarily off-limits; what it means is that it's important not to overindulge in them. Although we provide extensive lists of healthy, low-sodium choices in Appendix I (and some slightly higher-sodium foods in Appendix II) to make it easier for you to identify good food choices, we also want to teach you the basics so that you'll know how to read the labels for yourself and evaluate the claims of different food products.

Some foods are notorious for being high in sodium, such as chips, pretzels, and salted nuts. And most people know about the salt-laden reputation of canned soup and frozen entrees. Fewer people realize that processed meat, bacon, and sausage also contain loads of sodium. There are many foods that fill the grocery store shelves and freezers and are served at restaurants and fast-food chains that have just as much, if not more, salt than the "salty" foods you already know about. Let's start with what you find in the supermarket.

Supermarket Stroll

Take a stroll down the bread and cereal aisle and you'll find hundreds of options. You pick up a package of 100 percent whole-wheat bread thinking this is a really healthy choice, but when you read the label you see one slice has 240 milligrams of sodium. That may not sound too bad, but have two slices and you're already closing in on a quarter of your daily 2,300-milligram salt quota. That's *before* filling your sandwich with protein, let alone condiments. Likewise, the sodium in one 4-ounce packaged bagel—often 400 milligrams (if not more)—is nothing to sneeze at. You're probably wondering how anyone can stick to 2,300 milligrams of sodium per day, let alone the 1,500

Ten percent of the sodium we consume is naturally occurring in the food we eat, and the saltshaker contributes another 15 to 25 percent. The problem lies in processed foods and meals eaten away from home, which account for 65 to 75 percent of our sodium intake. Yup, you read that correctly—more than two-thirds of the salt in the average American diet comes from the processed foods that we buy at the grocery stores or the meals we eat in restaurants.

milligram limit of the Jumpstart Plan. Don't panic; you'll learn to spot the winners on the grocery shelves, and we've listed many of the best options for you in Appendix I.

Next take a look at the cereals. Some cereals, such as Rice Krispies and Raisin Bran, contain over 300 milligrams of sodium per serving—again, a lot of sodium to get from a single serving. You're in luck, though. Other cereals, such as Kashi Go Lean and regular instant oatmeal (see List A in Appendix I for other examples), have less than 100 milligrams of sodium per serving, only one-third the amount.

When buying dairy products, we're sure you're aware to look for low-fat versions, but did you ever stop to think about the sodium content of these foods? Most people don't, because they don't think of dairy foods as sodium-filled traps. But an ounce of sliced cheese typically has 100 to over 300 milligrams of sodium—and who stops at just one ounce? Think that's bad? One-half cup of cottage cheese, regardless of its fat content, can have from 300 to 450 milligrams of sodium.

Buying canned food is another area of caution. One cup of canned soup or half of a bouillon cube can have up to 1,000 milligrams of sodium, and a pack of dehydrated soup mix will rack up over 3,000 milligrams—more sodium than you should have in an entire day! Take a look at the canned vegetables, and you'll see why it's highly recommended to go for the frozen variety or the fresh stuff. Half a cup of canned spinach has 360 milligrams of sodium, whereas the same amount of frozen spinach has 173 milligrams—less than half as much. You can find an even bigger difference in other vegetables, such as asparagus. Five asparagus spears in a can have 430 milligrams of sodium, versus the 7.5 milligrams in the frozen variety, and *no* sodium in fresh spears. Now that's a sodium savings!

But before you start thinking that everything in the freezer aisle is better than the canned aisle, take a look at some of the sodium-filled culprits lurking behind the freezer doors. Looking for a sandwich to microwave and go? Think twice before you settle for one of those sodium-filled pockets. They have anywhere from 350 to 700 milligrams of sodium, not to mention the 16-plus grams of fat, at least 5 grams of which are saturated. Craving Chinese food? The restaurant varieties of dumplings and spring rolls may be bad for you, but the frozen options aren't much better. Six dumplings weigh in with over 600 milligrams of sodium—and that's not even with dipping sauce! If you don't have time to cook dinner or lunch, you may think you're making a good choice by eating a frozen meal rather than heading out to the nearest restaurant. Unfortunately most of those small, square boxes of low-fat entrees contain more sodium than you would expect for something seemingly "healthy." Want to save money and stock your freezer but skip the sodium and fat? Stick with frozen fruits and vegetables—they'll provide you with the vitamins and minerals you really need.

When shopping for condiments, keep in mind that you may have the healthiest meal in your salad bowl, but when you add the fixings it can all go downhill fast. Two tablespoons of a regular Italian dressing provide you with 120 calories, 13 grams of fat, and 400 milligrams of sodium. Think the "light" version will be better? Sadly, there's not much of a difference when it comes to the sodium. Two tablespoons of the light version will give you 60 calories, 6 grams of fat, and anywhere from 360 to 500 milligrams of sodium. You may get half the calories and fat, but not half the sodium. Sauces such as teriyaki, soy, barbecue, and tomato will leave you with more bloat than you ever want unless you learn how to become a label sleuth.

Nutrition Facts

Serving Size 1 cup (228g)
Servings Per Container 2

Amount Per Serving

Calories 250	Calories from Fat 110

	% Daily Value*
Total Fat 12g	18%
Saturated Fat 3g	15%
Trans Fat 1.5g	
Cholesterol 30mg	10%
Sodium 470mg	20%
Total Carbohydrate 31g	10%
Dietary Fiber 0g	0%
Sugars 5g	
Protein 5g	

Vitamin A	4%
Vitamin C	2%
Calcium	20%
Iron	4%

* Percent Daily Values are based on a 2,000 calorie diet. Your Daily Values may be higher or lower depending on your calorie needs:

	Calories:	2,000	2,500
Total Fat	Less than	65g	80g
Sat Fat	Less than	20g	25g
Cholesterol	Less than	300mg	300mg
Sodium	Less than	2,400mg	2,400mg
Total Carbohydrate		300g	375g
Dietary Fiber		25g	30g

Becoming Label Savvy

The number-one thing you can do to prevent sodium overconsumption is to read labels. The Nutrition Facts label on food packages tells you how much sodium is in one serving. There are a couple of things to keep in mind when looking at that sodium number. First, if the serving size is not the size you would usually eat, make sure you increase (or decrease) the amount of sodium according to the number of servings you intend to eat. For example, if the serving size listed on a package of bread is "one slice," and the label shows 240 milligrams of sodium, the sodium content of two slices of bread is 480 milligrams (240 milligrams per slice x 2 slices).

Next, the amount of sodium in a food may not mean much to you if you don't know what an appropriate amount is for that food, but if you compare similar foods to each other you will be able to make an informed decision. Let's go back to the bread example. If you look at two packages of bread side by side, and one package has 240 milligrams of sodium per slice and another has 140 milligrams, you know which one is a better choice when it comes to sodium content. But don't forget to look at the other important factors on the food label before making your purchase: calories, total fat, saturated fat, fiber, sugar, and the ingredient list.

When it comes to ingredients, here are some "red flag" items you should watch out for:

- Baking soda
- Baking powder
- Disodium phosphate
- Monosodium glutamate (MSG)
- Sodium alginate
- Sodium nitrate or nitrite

After checking out the serving size on the label, look to see if the product has a health claim on the package. Many foods these days claim to be "trans fat free" or "high in fiber." Some of the claims are regulated by the Food and Drug Administration (FDA), which means that they have specific definitions, which you should know before buying a product that bears a claim that just sounds good. Other claims are made by the food manufacturers and have no regulation behind them—this is why looking at all of the information provided (the

Nutrition Facts panel and the ingredients) is so important. Some claims that are specific to sodium are listed in the following chart along with their definitions. We are huge fans of the first four on this list, and you will be too! It's your immediate clue that a food meets at least one of the important slimming criteria.

Claim	What It Means
Sodium Free, Salt Free	Less than 5 milligrams of sodium per serving
Very Low Sodium	35 milligrams of sodium or less per serving
Low-Sodium	140 milligrams of sodium or less per serving
Unsalted, Without Added Salt, or No Salt Added	No salt is added during processing although the food usually is processed with salt.
Light in Sodium/Lightly Salted	At least 50 percent less sodium per serving than the average or reference amount for the same food with no sodium reduction
Reduced or Less Sodium	At least 25 percent less sodium per serving than the average reference amount for the same food with no sodium reduction

Look for these claims on the foods you buy, and you can be sure they will be lower in sodium than other foods that do not have the claims. But notice the "Reduced or Less Sodium" label claim. Don't be fooled. This isn't much better than the original product. For instance, a slice of turkey may have 400 milligrams of sodium. Its reduced-sodium counterpart would still have 300 milligrams—nowhere near the amount you'd find in a low-sodium food.

Other words to beware of when looking at the foods you are about to buy include "brined," "cured," "marinated," "pickled," and "smoked."

All of these terms imply that the food is salty. A quick check of the Nutrition Facts panel will likely confirm these are Red-Light Bloaters.

The perfect way to lower your salt intake when you're at the supermarket is to buy more fresh and frozen fruits and vegetables. Just be sure not to get the frozen vegetable with cheese or sauce packets. Fresh and frozen fruits and vegetables have less sodium than the canned varieties, plus they contain amazing minerals such as potassium and magnesium that help offset the sodium you take in. If you must get something from the canned food aisle, look for the low-sodium or unsalted varieties. Keep these other tips in mind when you're at the grocery store:

- **Buy fewer prepared foods**—the less processing, the less sodium.
- **Be choosy about your cheese**—look first for low-fat, then low-sodium varieties, younger cheeses like mozzarella, and ones without added flavors.
- **Pick your deli meats carefully**—some of them can have 800 milligrams of sodium or more in just a few slices. Look for low-sodium ones, which should have less than 350 milligrams for 2 ounces. Otherwise, look for those with less than 480 milligrams of sodium for 2 ounces.
- **Buy soup ingredients, not soup**—unless you can find a low-sodium variety since premade soup contains a lot more sodium than you would add on your own (see Soups in Appendix II). Buy the vegetables and low-sodium stock, and add the flavorings yourself.

If you find that you're having a hard time identifying foods that are low in sodium, try looking at the percent Daily Value (DV) on the Nutrition Facts panel. The Daily Values (DV) are a set of reference values based on the RDA (Recommended Dietary Allowances) developed by the FDA specifically for food labeling. They are a sort of one-size-fits-all recommendation, designed to help you plan a healthy diet. Aim to select foods that have 5 percent or less DV for sodium per serving.

Here are some more helpful sodium swaps:

Instead of:	Choose:
Smoked, cured, salted, and canned meat, fish, and poultry	Fresh or frozen meat, fish, and poultry
Regular peanut butter or natural peanut butter with salt	Low-sodium peanut butter or natural peanut butter without salt
Salted crackers	Unsalted crackers
Regular canned and dehydrated soups, broths, and bouillons	Low-sodium canned soups, broths, and bouillons
Regular canned vegetables	Fresh and frozen vegetables
Salted snack foods	Unsalted or lightly salted chips, pretzels, popcorn, etc.
Salted butter	Unsalted butter or whipped butter; better yet: butter spray
High-salt salad dressings	Oil and vinegar with lemon and/or herbs; Wishbone Salad Spritzers; 1 teaspoon of grated Parmesan cheese; specialty vinegars; lemon and pepper

Fast-Food Shuffle

If you think the amount of sodium in packaged foods at the super-market is frightening, brace yourself—fast-food and restaurant favorites are the real doozies. Below we have listed entrees found at popular fast-food, take-out, and chain restaurants. Some may sound healthy (others not so much), but look closely at the nutrition information and you'll see why you should rethink your order the next time you head out for food on the run.

Fast-Food Sodium Saboteurs

Chipotle Mexican Grill Chicken Burrito ....1,179 calories; 47 grams fat; 2,656 milligrams sodium

Quiznos Classic Italian Sandwich (large) .....1,528 calories; 92 grams fat; 4,604 milligrams sodium

Uno Chicago Grill Classic Deep Dish Pizza
(individual pie) ....2,310 calories; 162 grams fat; 4,470 milligrams sodium

Macaroni Grill Calamari Fritti ....1,210 calories; 78 grams fat; 4,170 milligrams sodium

Macaroni Grill Spaghetti and Meatballs
with Meat Sauce ....2,430 calories; 128 grams fat; 5,290 milligrams sodium

On the Border Grande Fajita Nachos with
Mesquite-Grilled Chicken (appetizer) ....1,890 calories; 113 grams fat; 3,790 milligrams sodium

McDonald's Bacon, Egg, and Cheese
Biscuit (large) ....520 calories; 30 grams fat; 1,520 milligrams sodium

Subway Cold Cut Combo (6-inch) ....410 calories; 17 grams fat; 1,530 milligrams sodium

---

Many of the above items are a double-edged sword—they are high in sodium and fat. Many of these meals contain more calories than you should get in an entire day! Eat these foods and not only will your waistline expand from fat and bloat, but your blood pressure and cholesterol will rise to levels you don't want to see. Even fast-food items such as Chili's Guiltless Chicken Sandwich, with only 490 calories and 8 grams of fat, and Boston Market's white BBQ chicken, with 340 calories and 11 grams of fat, still have 2,720 and 1,270 milligrams of sodium, respectively—not so guiltless, after all, when you keep in mind that you should get no more than 2,300 milligrams of sodium a day (and only 1,500 during the Jumpstart Plan). So what can you do to make up for some of the damage done if you eat these sodium monstrosities in a moment of weakness? We've got the answers!

Quick-Fix Cures for a Salt Hangover

The day after Chinese takeout you step on the scale and you've put on three pounds. You feel bloated, your fingers are puffy, and you have bags under your eyes. You have what we call a "salt hangover." Next time, try one of these remedies:

Emergency Salt Hangover Remedies

❑ Drink at least 2 cups of water—one with the fresh-squeezed juice of $1/2$ lemon and the other with the fresh-squeezed juice of $1/4$ orange. The water will flush out the excess sodium along with the water the sodium is holding onto. The fresh lemon and orange juice provide a hefty boost of potassium that will flush the salt even faster. *(Count as 2 Beverage Slimmers)*

❑ Drink 2 cups of green tea and eat 4 Sunsweet Dried Plums *(Count as 2 Beverage Slimmers and 1 Flusher/Anti-Bloaters [Fruit])*

❑ Mix a batch of The Nutrition Twins Salt Detox Juice. Thoroughly blend the following ingredients together, ideally in a juicer: 3 sprigs parsley (parsley is a natural diuretic); 6 carrots, scrubbed well and tops removed; $1/2$ beet (optional); 1 red or yellow apple, cored and seeds removed. Makes 2 servings. *(Count as 3 Flushers/Anti-Bloaters [$1/2$ Fruit])*

❑ Drink 2 cups of our Salt Detox Juice or 2 cups of green tea and eat 1 cup steamed spinach spritzed with juice from a lemon. Spinach is packed with potassium to flush the excess salt along with the lemon. The fiber in the spinach will help push plugging foods out of the colon and slim down a bloated belly. *(Count as 2 Beverage Slimmers, 2 Flushers/Anti-Bloaters)*

❑ Try The Nutrition Twins Tea and Melon Cure. Drink 2 cups of tea (peppermint, ginger, chamomile, and/or fennel tea [these are all digestive enhancers]); eat 1 cup of cubed cantaloupe, 1 cup of melon, or 1 cup of watermelon. *(Count as 2 Beverage Slimmers, 1 Flusher/Anti-Bloater [Fruit])*

❑ Drink 2 cups of tea with lemon, and eat 4 dried plums and 30 unsalted pistachios. Pistachios are the skinny nut. They're one of the lowest in fat, highest in protein, and highest in fiber, which means they are one of the few protein sources that have fiber to help unplug you while satiating you. *(Count as 1 Mono Slimmer, 1 Flusher/Anti-Bloater, 2 Beverage Slimmers.)*

Cooking at Home

When eating at home, first things first: take the saltshaker out of the equation. If you are cooking a meal starting from scratch with completely unprocessed, wholesome foods, occasionally using some kosher salt while cooking is okay, just don't overdo it; remember to taste as you cook. Note that some of our recipes that are used in the Jumpstart menu plans contain salt; however, this is factored into the total recipe and the sodium remains low. When you use delicious spices, you'll usually find that you don't need to add salt at all. If you must use salt, limit it to ⅛ teaspoon (ideally kosher or sea salt) per serving, as this equals 300 milligrams in table salt (and less in kosher or sea salt). This means that a meal comprising unprocessed food and ⅛ tablespoon of salt will easily fall below 600 milligrams of sodium per meal, which will help to ensure that you consume less than 2,300 milligrams of sodium a day. Just keep in mind that anytime you're adding salt to your cooking, it's hard to tell whether a dish has enough flavoring until the flavors have melded together for a long enough period of time. While you can always add more salt, you can't take extra out. So add salt at the end of cooking—you will likely taste the salt when the food first touches your tongue, and that salty taste will carry through to the rest of your bites. In this way, you'll avoid taking in extra sodium and still get the salty taste you love.

Salt 101

Table Salt: Table salt is the most common salt. It's what's in the saltshaker at a restaurant and what you most likely use to add flavor to your food at a meal. Table salt typically comes from rock salt and is mined from underground salt mineral deposits. It's then fully refined into pure sodium chloride, without the remnants of any other minerals.

Sea Salt: Another common salt, sea salt is produced from evaporated seawater—not the cheapest means of production, hence the hefty price tag. Sea salt tends to have small amounts of other minerals besides sodium and chloride, such as calcium and magnesium, which is why it has a slightly different taste from table salt and can vary in color. Although sea salt can be completely refined like table salt, it is most often left unrefined, which is why it has bigger crystals than table salt.

Many companies boast that their products that contain sea salt have less sodium than others made with more refined salts. Does sea salt really have less sodium than table salt? Yes and no. Sea salt has bigger grains than table salt, so teaspoon for teaspoon sea salt will have less sodium. Think of it as pebbles versus sand. A bucket of pebbles will weigh less than a bucket of sand because there's more space and air between the pebbles than between the grains of sand. Similarly, a teaspoon of sea salt will weigh less than a teaspoon of table salt because the crystals are bigger and there's more air between them. So while 1 teaspoon of sea salt has about 1,900 milligrams of sodium, 1 teaspoon of table salt has about 2,400 milligrams of sodium. However, an equal *weight* of sea salt and table salt have equal amounts of sodium. That said, sea salt is often a better choice; people who use it generally consume less sodium because they use less of it and they use it differently. Because sea salt loses its flavor in the cooking process, it is usually added to food at the end of cooking. That way the flavor is more immediate to the taste buds, and a little bit goes a longer way than with table salt, which more readily dissolves in food.

Kosher Salt: Kosher salt can come from mines or seawater, but what makes it different from table salt and sea salt is that it is "raked" during evaporation. The raking process is what gives kosher salt its coarse grains. Even though kosher salt was designed to be used for the preparation of kosher meats, many chefs and home cooks use kosher salt for all their cooking because of the ease of use. The coarse grains make it easy to measure by touch and toss into pots and pans. And kosher salt sticks to food better than other varieties of salt because of its larger surface area. So you can use it to make a salt crust on meat and fish (the crust comes right off when it's done, so it's a great way to bake these proteins without adding a lot of fat and salt to the actual food) and for preserving and pickling food. Like sea salt, teaspoon per teaspoon, kosher salt has less sodium than table salt—again, because of its bigger crystals.

Many recipes that use salt call for salt "to taste," which means it's really in your hands to choose how much you want to add. For those recipes that call for a specific amount, remember that you can reduce that amount or completely remove it from the recipe without compromising flavor. To add flavor without adding salt, why not try fresh herbs and spices? They'll give your taste buds something new to experience. Onion and garlic (and their powders), thyme, rosemary, basil, cumin, and cinnamon are just few. Add flavor by using fresh lemons or lemon juice, vinegar and wine. No matter what you use in place of salt, remember to have fun with it and experiment.

Seasoning with Slimming Spices

Savory flavors and seasonings with "bite" are the most effective in replacing the taste of salt. Examples include:

Basil	Cumin	Garlic powder
Black pepper	Curry powder	Ginger
Coriander	Dill seeds	Onion powder

Use the "powdered" form of garlic and onion, *not* the "salt" form.

Omit the salt when cooking pasta and flavor the sauce with basil, oregano, parsley, and pepper, or use an Italian seasoning blend. As a general rule, add *fresh* herbs near the end of cooking or just before serving. Prolonged heating can cause flavor and aroma losses. The more delicate fresh herbs can be added a minute or two before the end of cooking or sprinkled on food before serving. Examples of delicate herbs include basil, chives, cilantro, and dill leaves. Less delicate fresh herbs can be added during the last 20 minutes of cooking. Examples include: dill seeds, rosemary, tarragon, and thyme. *Whole* dried spices and herbs (such as whole allspice and bay leaves) release flavors more slowly than crumbled or ground ones. They are ideal for dishes cooking an hour or more, such as soups and stews.

Food	Spice It Up With:
Vegetables	
Asparagus	Black pepper, garlic powder, lemon, nutmeg, vinegar
Broccoli	Basil, black pepper, garlic powder, lemon, onion, oregano
Brussels sprouts	Chestnut, lemon, marjoram, nutmeg, oregano, sage
Cabbage	Caraway, celery or poppy seeds, dry mustard, green pepper, onion, oregano, pimiento, vinegar
Carrots	Black pepper, chives, cinnamon, cloves, dill, garlic powder, ginger, lemon, marjoram, mint, nutmeg, rosemary, sage, thyme
Cauliflower	Basil, chives, lemon, nutmeg, paprika, parsley, rosemary
Collard, kale, mustard, or turnip greens	Garlic powder, lemon, onions, oregano, parsley, vinegar
Corn	Cumin, curry powder, onion powder, paprika, parsley
Cucumbers	Basil, dill, lemon, oregano, vinegar

Food *(continued)*	Spice It Up With:
Eggplant	Basil, chives, garlic powder, lemon, onion, oregano, parsley, tarragon
Green beans	Basil, celery, curry powder, dill, garlic powder, lemon, low-sodium bouillon powder, marjoram, nutmeg, onions, oregano, pimiento, tarragon, thyme
Greens	Black pepper, onion
Okra	Bay leaf, black pepper, lemon, thyme
Onions	Garlic powder, green pepper, nutmeg, red pepper
Potatoes	Dill, garlic powder, onion powder, paprika, parsley, sage
Summer squash	Dill, garlic powder, onion powder, paprika, parsley, sage
Tomatoes	Basil, bay leaf, black pepper, celery, curry, dill, garlic powder, marjoram, onion powder, oregano, parsley, sage, savory, thyme
Winter Squash	Cinnamon, ginger, nutmeg, onion powder
Meat, Poultry, and Fish	
Beef	Bay leaf, black pepper, marjoram, nutmeg, onion powder, sage, thyme
Pork	Black pepper, garlic powder, onion powder, oregano, sage
Poultry	Ginger, marjoram, oregano, paprika, poultry seasoning, rosemary, sage, tarragon, thyme
Fish	Black pepper, curry powder, dill, dry mustard, marjoram, paprika

Eating Out

When you're practicing being salt-savvy, things get a little tougher when you dine out. First, watch the bread basket. We know—warm, crusty rolls or soft sourdough can really be enticing, but the amount of sodium (not to mention the calories) can wreak havoc on your body. If you can't live without the bread basket, indulge in one slice, preferably whole grain, and push the rest away. The bread adds hundreds of calories to your day, especially when it's dipped in oil or butter.

 Before going out to eat, have a warm cup of tea and some vegetables. This "pre-meal" is virtually calorie-free and will prevent you from feeling ravenous when you get to the restaurant; you'll be able to pass on the bread and make a rational, healthy decision about what you are going to order.

Next up: ordering your meal. Don't be shy about asking your server how dishes are prepared. Order the entree grilled, baked, broiled, poached, steamed, or roasted. You can also ask them not to add salt (or ask for a minimal amount of salt, at least until your taste buds adjust).

Avoid ordering foods that are smoked, fried, breaded, pickled, cured, stuffed, basted, or "au gratin," "a la king," "alfredo," or "parmagiana"— these are all major Flabbers (see chapter 8). Also watch out for any sauces that contain soy sauce, teriyaki sauce, gravy, or broth—all Bloaters.

When dining out at Japanese restaurants where soy sauce is standard, ask for reduced-sodium soy and use it sparingly—you'll avoid at least 350 milligrams of sodium. Be aware that just a teaspoon of the reduced-sodium variety will still cost you almost 200 milligrams of sodium.

Just as we recommend you do at home, don't use the saltshaker; use the pepper instead. Ask for condiments, such as mustard, ketchup, pickles, sauerkraut, olives, and salt-filled sauces, on the side, so that you can control how much you have—and then only have a little bit! If you order a salad, ask for oil and vinegar or vinaigrette (better yet, just balsamic vinegar or lemon) on the side, in place of creamy dressings. In the mood for soup? Once again, ask about the preparation. Many broth- and tomato-based soups are very high in sodium, and creamy soups usually are high in fat. When it comes to side dishes, opt for fresh vegetables—have them steamed to save your waistline, and make sure no extra salt (or butter/oil) is added. For dessert, stick with fresh fruit or sorbet—you'll save calories, fat, and sodium.

Now that you've learned how to be salt savvy, you should feel *nearly* unstoppable. You know how to handle almost any situation—whether you are cooking, at a restaurant, heading to a cocktail party, or salt-overloaded. Chapter 5 gives you the tools to put the final pieces of the slimming puzzle together—portion size guidance, being held account-able, and learning your eating and overeating cues—this will make your salt- and fat-slashing journey that much easier.

Tools to Keep You On Track: The Rule of the Hand and the Food Log

We live in a supersized society where everything from beverages to snacks to bagels is overstuffed. In fact, restaurant portions are so enormous that they distort our perception; it's often hard to tell what a normal serving size looks like. Prevent "portion distortion" by measuring out ½ cup and 1 cup of cooked pasta or rice and placing each portion on a plate so that you can visualize exactly what those servings look like. This doesn't mean that you can eat only a ½-cup or 1-cup serving at each meal, but it will give you a realistic idea of what those servings look like and remind you of how quickly they can accumulate. Repeating this exercise frequently will remind you what "normal" really is and help you keep portions under control.

Most people would describe their lives as hectic. Since the majority of Americans eat at least one meal per day away from home, using measuring utensils to portion food is not always an option. What's more, restaurant plates are often not the same size as those at the home, which can exacerbate portion distortion. But you can still eat the right portions and lose weight by using our Rule of Hand.

The Rule of Hand

Your hand, as surprising as it may sound, plays a critical role when it comes to your weight loss and dream body. Your hand is with you wherever you go, and it will help you estimate portion sizes.

Use the following equivalents to judge food quantities without a measuring cup:

Food that fits in the cup of your hand = 1/2 cup

A woman's fist = 1 cup

A man's fist = 1 1/2 cups

3 fingers = 2 ounces of lean meat

While paying attention to portion sizes is important, so is paying attention to the volume of food you're eating, which is why a food journal is a great tool for you on your weight-loss journey.

The Food Log

As simple as it may sound, one of the best ways to guarantee your success on any eating plan is to keep a journal, also known as a food diary. Tracking what you eat holds you accountable for your actions. We have clients who tell us that when they keep a record of what they eat, they eat less, if only because they don't feel like writing down each and every morsel that passes their lips (the one time that laziness pays off). What's more, our clients say it makes them aware of what they are actually eating. When you first see the list of foods that you have consumed in a day, it can be shocking.

Awareness, Acceptance, Accountability

By tracking what you eat, you will see how your behavior compares to your intentions. For example, it's easy to eat several cookies and "forget" or pretend it never happened. However, journaling encourages you to be honest with yourself. Writing it down forces you to accept the truth that, yes, you *did* eat those cookies. When we don't write down what we eat, it's easy *not* to hold ourselves accountable, to not do what we claim *we really want* to do. Instead, we abandon our good intentions and fudge it, finding legitimate-sounding excuses, reasons, explanations, or rationalizations for wiggling out of our commitment to ourselves. Sure, we say we want to eat well, lose weight, safeguard our health, honor our body, and save the planet. Then life intervenes; we get distracted by stress, temptations, fatigue, and convenience: "It would be just so easy to microwave a pizza for dinner right now!" We find ways to have what we want when we want it, then find ways to explain and justify our choices. This happens on both a conscious and unconscious level, and it can be a challenge to catch ourselves in the act. And if we don't write it down, well, in our mind, maybe it just didn't happen. . . .

Do these sound familiar?

"This is the first thing I've eaten all day."

"I've been so 'good' lately; I deserve this."

"No, I didn't eat that last brownie. Uh-uh, wasn't me."

"I don't understand why I can't lose weight/why I gain weight/why I'm so bloated."

"The elliptical machine said I burned 750 calories today; I can have seconds."

"I had a horrid day—I earned this bacon cheeseburger!"

"I had no time, so I stopped at the drive-through."

"Have all you want—olive oil is good for you!"

"It's organic/low fat/low sodium/sugar-free/whole wheat."

"But it's my birthday/the holidays/a celebration! I must have some cake/pie/dessert!"

We may be able to trick to ourselves into thinking we really followed our healthy goals, but we won't be able to fool the scale or our tight-fitting clothes.

This is your opportunity to stop yourself in your tracks before you sabotage yourself. How? By coming clean and writing it all down. It's that simple. Our clients keep a detailed food log of everything—yes, we mean *everything*—that they eat every day. Yes, every day. And they do this until they don't need to do it to stay on track. If they ever start to feel themselves slip, they start keeping their food diary again to get them back on track and to keep them slim. Writing everything includes the two sugars and milk in your latte, three times a day; the peanut butter you eat out of the jar when you prepare your kids' lunches; the bag of M&M'S that gets you through your usual 4:00 PM slump; the mouthful after mouthful of pasta you sample as you prepare dinner, in addition to the pasta you put on your plate; the handfuls of chips you munch over margaritas; and of course, the margaritas (which contain sugar, salt, and alcohol and can have over 1,000 calories!). We're not talking just your Slimmers; we're talking *everything*.

A 2008 study by Kaiser Permanente found that those people who write down what they eat lose twice as much weight as those who don't. Just another reason to pick up that pen.

Food journaling will help you discover those "aha" moments as you become aware of habits that are holding you back from your weight-loss goals. Sure, we eat when we're hungry, but very often we also eat when we're bored, when we're upset, when something pushes our buttons and triggers a craving, when it's "time to eat," when we think we deserve a reward, or when we need to escape. Keeping a food journal lets you identify what, when, where, and why you eat and puts you back in control. As a result of recording your food choices, you may be shocked by:

- The sheer quantity of food you consume in a day
- The poor food choices you make, habitually and/or spontaneously, time and time again
- The people and events that trigger cravings and/or bingeing
- How easily people, activities, availability, and other factors influence you

The eating patterns that are revealed when you keep a journal may also surprise you. For example:

- You automatically reach for those salty, crunchy chips whenever you feel stressed or angry.
- The Chinese food you take out three times a week gives you heartburn and keeps you up at night.
- You feel sluggish, bloated, and depressed after you indulge in pepperoni pizza, your favorite splurge.
- All those half-cup refills of coffee add up to over 6 cups a day.
- More often than not, one cocktail turns into three, sometimes four.

With a better *awareness* of your food choices and *acceptance* of how great an impact they have upon your body and mind, heart and soul, you will seize the opportunity to take control of your actions. Rather than default to past patterns, or fall victim to events, people, and circumstances, show up on the page and hold yourself *accountable*. Take control of your diet; become lean, bloat-free, and happy.

What, When, Where, How Much, Why, and Who

To assist you in your journaling efforts, we've designed a convenient Food Log to make the process nearly effortless (see page 285). You can make copies of this log so that you'll have one for each day of the week.

You'll record Slimmers, Bloaters, Flushers, and everything else you eat—and you'll be able to see how you stack up against your goal. You'll also track the amount of water and tea you drink each day, what times you eat, how hungry you are before and after eating, and what mood you are in. Reviewing your Food Log will lead to those all-important "aha" moments. For example, you may realize that you overeat whenever you're angry or that you're resistant to drinking enough water during the day. These "aha" moments are the motivating force you need to lose weight.

Discovering Your Questionable Bloaters

For some people, specific foods and beverages create a distended stomach even though they don't increase body fat or contain high amounts of sodium. We call these "Questionable Bloaters."

Questionable Bloaters

Carbonated Beverages such as seltzer and diet sodas (Note: Diet soda shouldn't be consumed liberally, even if it doesn't bloat you. It should be limited to no more than one, 12-ounce serving daily.) These drinks can fill you up with air and cause stomach distention.

Sugar substitutes like sorbitol, xylitol, maltitol, isomalt, lactitol, mannitol, erythritol, and hydrogenated starch hydrolysates (HSH): These are sugar alcohols and may be found in any food labeled "sugar-free." Check ingredient labels.

Sugar alcohols are slowly and only partially digested, lingering in your gut where your body's bacteria feed on them, resulting in gas. If you're lucky, you may hardly even notice this, but others may have just two pieces of sugar-free candy and want to hide out for the rest of the night.

To see if you are sensitive to these foods, simply eat or drink a food and use your journal to record your body's response (i.e. if you become excessively bloated). If you can eat Questionable Bloaters without feeling or looking bloated, then go ahead. If you are sensitive to these foods, test your level of tolerance by consuming a very small amount (1/4 cup of seltzer or 1 sugar-free candy with malitol) to see if you have a limit to what your body can tolerate while remaining symptom-free. For instance, 1/2 cup of seltzer may not bother you, but 2/3 cup may leave you feeling like you could float out of the room.

The first Food Log column allows you to record the time that you eat each meal and snack. This will keep you aware of how long it has been since you last ate. Eating too often may signal that you are turning to food to satisfy an emotional need, while waiting too long may set you up to binge or overeat because you are feeling ravenous.

Most people are out of touch with their sense of hunger. The second column helps you to gain the power to control your weight by recognizing and measuring how hungry you are before you eat and how full you are after you've eaten. Each time you sit down to eat (and you *should* be sitting down when you eat), make a note of your hunger. Relearn your feelings of hunger and satiety by noting in your Log how hungry you are on a scale of 1

Are Artificial Sweeteners Safe?
The American Dietetic Association (ADA) believes consumers can safely enjoy a range of nutritive and nonnutritive sweeteners (in moderation, of course!). Keeping your food journal will reveal rare instances when such sweeteners cause stomach distress for sensitive individuals.

(Thanksgiving Day full/overstuffed) to 10 (feeling as if you haven't eaten in days/starving) before each meal and then immediately after you eat. If you finish a meal and rate your level of fullness as a "1," you know you are eating too much. This is why you should check in with your level of fullness halfway through your meal, as it should help you to gauge how hungry you are feeling.

Does the environment play a role in weight management? Absolutely! The next column in the Food Log allows you to see if you mindlessly munch and end up overeating in front of the TV, the refrigerator, or the cupboard. No matter where you eat—whether it's with friends, alone in a quiet, candlelit room, or with family in a bright, noisy place—the atmosphere affects everything from your mood, to what you eat, to how much and how fast you eat. Eating quickly doesn't allow you to fully enjoy your meal. It takes twenty minutes for your brain to receive the signal that your stomach is satisfied, so you must allow this time to prevent overeating. Learn to recognize environments that negatively impact the foods and quantities you choose so that you can avoid or change them to aid your weight-loss success.

Use the remaining boxes on the food log to describe what you ate, and then write the number of servings of each food that you had in the appropriate category box. At the end of the day, add up your servings for each of the categories (Carbohydrate Slimmers, Protein Slimmers, etc.) to see how you compared to your goal. If you prefer not to count your servings, simply use the food diary to record what you eat and how you feel. Simply by journaling what you eat, you will feel much better as you are being proactive and taking the first step on your weight-loss crusade.

Chapter 6

Phase 2:
The Maintenance Plan

Congratulations! If you've made it this far, you have completed the Jumpstart Plan, and you're feeling great. You've lost pounds, and you're more sculpted, more energetic, and bloat-free. You're well on your way to achieving your dream body. As if this weren't enough, your taste buds have embarked on their journey of taste-bud turnover. This means in just a few more weeks your mouth will water for Slimmers, Flushers, and Anti-Bloaters, and your palate will have less tolerance for salt-laden foods that expand your waistline.

Although you may have lost 5 pounds or more during the Jumpstart phase, you can expect to lose 1 to 2 pounds of body fat a week during the Maintenance phase. This is a safe and healthy weight loss and will help to ensure long-lasting results.

On the Maintenance phase, you are permitted up to 2,300 milligrams of sodium instead of the 1,500 milligrams you were allowed during the Jumpstart Phase. For you calorie counters, women on the Maintenance Plan can have about 1,400 calories, and men can have 1,600 calories. The extra food during this phase will keep you satiated and help you feel strong as you cruise through your day. If you have a tendency to feel deprived and then binge, you may need an additional 150 to 200 calories daily (roughly 1.5 Carbohydrate Slimmer servings *or* 1.5 Protein Slimmer servings). But test this plan first to see if it satiates you before adding more food. On the other hand, if you have tried other weight-loss plans with little success, if you're a small female who seems to have a slow metabolism or a male with a small stature (about 5'5" or smaller), or you don't meet the minimum exercise requirements in Chapter 9 to get at least 30 minutes of activity (or at least some kind of movement) most days of the week, we recommend that you stick close to the same number of calories that you consumed during the Jumpstart phase to achieve optimum results. This means that although the Maintenance phase allows 2 daily servings of the Red Light foods (Pluggers, Bloaters, Flabbers, or Chubbers; see chapter 8), you should stick to just 1 Red Light food serving daily.

In an ideal world, we would all continue to eat only the slimming foods found in the Jumpstart Plan. However, in reality, this can be tough. And we want you to succeed—not just for ten days or eight weeks, but for good. So although you will still focus on the foods that you have been eating, phase 2 allows for more flexibility with the Slimmers, while also permitting Red Light foods—bloating and fatty foods—in portions small enough for you to still achieve your dream body. Note: If you choose to skip either of your two daily servings of the Red Light foods, you can have an extra Carbohydrate or Protein Slimmer serving for each that you forgo.

If you found that eating the foods in the Jumpstart phase was easy for you and worked well with your lifestyle, you can skip this chapter and continue to eat as you have been—only now allow yourself 2 daily servings of the Red Light foods (see Appendix III) or two additional Slimmers each day.

You'll find additions to the Carbohydrate, Protein, and Mono Slimmers categories in Appendix II. There is also a new category called Convenience Prepared Foods that offers even more flexibility to ensure success on your most hectic days. Convenience Prepared Foods are foods that require little, if any, preparation. We created this list because we are aware that not everyone will be able to eat fresh, wholesome Slimmers made from scratch at every meal. We have found many prepared foods that provide energizing and anti-aging nutrients and fiber with minimal amounts of sodium, calories, and chubbing fat. Some are pleasantly sur-prising—much less "flabbing" and bloating than you'd imagine—in fact, some are actually slimming. These Convenience Prepared Foods meet certain healthy criteria/qualifications (Table 3), and you will use calories as a guide to count them. Other Convenience Prepared Foods meet many of these healthy criteria, but lack one of the benefits; they are qual-ified as Yellow Light foods. Yellow Light foods are not as wholesome as the other Slimmers, but aren't as damaging as the Red Light Pluggers, Bloaters, Chubbers, or Flabbers, either. You can have *one* Yellow Light food a day; it will take the place of one of your Green-Light Slimmers. Generally, Yellow Light foods have more sodium than Green Light foods but less than 600 milligrams. They also have at least one redeem-ing quality. For instance, fat-free refried beans are a bit high in sodium, but they are high in fiber and nutrients. Similarly, white rice is con-sidered a Yellow Light food because although it's not a whole grain (it lacks fiber and other nutrients), it is fat free and practically sodium free.

That makes it lower in sodium than even most whole-grain breads. In Appendix II you'll find a list of Yellow Light Slimmers. You'll continue to combat any of the plugging that they may do by having a Flusher or an Anti-Bloater with them, as you do with all your meals.

You'll notice that Table 3 shows the same number of servings you had in the Jumpstart Plan, but also includes shaded areas that indicate the additions to the table. The additions include Yellow Light foods (one Yellow Light food can *replace* one Green Light Slimmer serving one time per day), 2 Red Light servings, and a condiment. Although you still get your 4 Freebies, you also now get a condiment, which has more calories and sodium than Freebies.

Table 3: Maintenance Plan Daily Servings
(Shaded Sections Indicate Additions After the Jumpstart Phase Is Completed)

	Servings per Day (Women)	Servings per Day (Men)
Carbohydrate Slimmers (List A Foods)	4	5
Protein Slimmers (List B Foods)	5 (at least 2 from Dairy)	6.5 (at least 2 from Dairy)
Mono Slimmers (List C Foods)	1	1
Flushers/Anti-Bloaters (List D Foods)	5–9 Vegetables (Work your way up to 9) 2 Fruits	5–10 Vegetables (Work your way up to 9 or 10) 2 Fruits
Beverage Slimmers (Water or Tea)	8+ (See page 41 for number of servings based on your weight.)	8+ (See page 41 for number of servings based on your weight.)
Freebies	4	4
Condiments	1	1

Table 3: Maintenance Plan Daily Servings *(continued)*

	Servings per Day (Women)	Servings per Day (Men)
Yellow Light Foods	1 (Must replace 1 Carb or Protein Slimmer) (If Yellow Light food has more than 100 calories, count first 100 as Yellow Light food and each additional 100 calories as a Slimmer.)	1 (Must replace 1 Carb or Protein Slimmer)
Red Light Foods (Pluggers, Bloaters, Chubbers, Flabbers)	2	2

In Table 4 to follow you'll see the sodium qualifications for Maintenance Plan foods as well as some of the characteristics these foods must have in order to be considered Green Light foods. (Yellow Light foods fall slightly outside these guidelines.) Just as in the Jumpstart phase, serving sizes for bread and cereals are based on their calories — a bread or cereal that is higher in calories must be counted as more than 1 Carbohydrate Slimmer serving (see specifics in Table 4).

Again, just as in the Jumpstart Plan, you'll create a slimming meal by choosing one food from List A, List B, and List D on Table 4. You can also choose an option from List C *once a day* and up to four condiment Freebies and one Condiment. You can still choose from the Brand-Name Green Light foods in Appendix I, but you'll now also have the brand-name options added in Appendix II. You can also have up to two servings of the Red Light foods listed in Appendix III. Table 4 lists the general guidelines for food categories, just as it did in the Jumpstart Phase, only now some areas are shaded to indicate additions and changes for the Maintenance phase.

Table 4: Slimmer Servings

Note: Foods with more sodium than Slimmers but less than 600 mg, count as 1 Yellow Light food (except grains and cereals).

Maintenance Food	Sodium Limit (2,300 mg a day)	Maintenance Slimmer Serving Qualifications	Count Each Serving As
CARBOHYDRATE SLIMMERS (List A Foods)			
Bread (whole grains only): wraps, pita, English muffins, other whole grains like popcorn	≤200 mg/ per serving	≤120 calories ≥2 grams fiber	1 Carbohydrate Slimmer
	≤275 mg/ per serving	121–150 calories ≥2 grams fiber	1.5 Carbohydrate Slimmers
	≤350 mg/ per serving	151–200 calories ≥2 grams fiber	2 Carbohydrate Slimmers
Whole-Grain Pasta, Brown Rice	≤100 mg/ per serving	≤120 calories ≥2 grams fiber	1 Carbohydrate Slimmer
Cereal: Whole grain only—first label ingredient should say "whole"	≤200 mg/ per serving	≤120 calories ≤8 grams sugar ≥5 grams fiber (≥3 grams fiber if hot cereal)	1 Carbohydrate Slimmer
	≤275 mg/ per serving	121–150 calories ≤12 grams sugar ≥5 grams fiber (≥3 grams fiber if hot cereal)	1.5 Carbohydrate Slimmers
	≤350 mg/ per serving	151–200 calories ≤16 grams sugar ≥5 grams fiber (≥3 grams fiber if hot cereal)	2 Carbohydrate Slimmers
Starchy Vegetables, Starchy Tomato Sauce, Beans, fresh or canned/processed *(Note: You can count beans as a Carbohydrate Slimmer or a Protein Slimmer)*	≤240 mg/ per serving	50–100 calories Rinse all beans and vegetables	1 Carbohydrate Slimmer
	241 mg–600 mg	50–100 calories, Rinse all beans and vegetables	1 Yellow Light Food

Maintenance Food	Sodium Limit (2,300 mg a day)	Maintenance Slimmer Serving Qualifications	Count Each Serving As
PROTEIN SLIMMERS (List B Foods)			
Cheese, Milk (and Soy Milk), and Dairy products (Nonfat and Low-fat only)	≤240 mg/ per serving (cottage cheese: limit to one, ≤400 mg per ½-cup serving per day)	≤3 grams fat per serving Yogurt (6-ounce serving): ≤100 calories, ≤1 gram saturated fat, ≤30 grams added sugar (12 grams occurs naturally), ≥20% of DV for calcium. (Greek yogurt: ≤10% DV calcium.) Soy Milk: ≤100 calories per serving. Yogurt: same qualifications as above with 101–140 calories per serving	1 Protein Slimmer (Dairy serving) 1.5 Protein Slimmers (Dairy)
Meat, Poultry, Tofu, Tempeh	≤140 mg if single raw ingredient/ 2 ounce	Choose only skinless poultry breast, beef round or loin, or pork tenderloin (limit beef and pork to twice a week)	1 Protein Slimmer
All Fish and Seafood including Clams, Oysters, Scallops, Shrimp, Squid (aka Calamari), Mussels, Crab, and Lobster	Limit sodium to ≤240 mg per 2-ounce raw ingredient	Limit mussels and lobster to twice a week Limit crab to once a week	1 Protein Slimmer
Canned Fish and Poultry	≤240 mg per 2 ounces canned 241–600 mg sodium		1 Protein Slimmer 1 Yellow Light Food
Deli Meats	≤480 mg per 2-once serving	Stick to one, 2-ounce serving or count second serving as a Yellow Light Food	1 Protein Slimmer
	480–600 mg per serving	Stick to one, 2-ounce serving	Yellow Light Food

Maintenance Food	Sodium Limit (2,300 mg a day)	Maintenance Slimmer Serving Qualifications	Count Each Serving As
PROTEIN SLIMMERS (List B Foods) *continued*			
Beans: dried, canned/processed (Note: You can count beans as a Carbohydrate Slimmer or a Protein Slimmer)	≤ 240 sodium per serving 241–600 mg per serving	All canned beans should be rinsed	1 Protein Slimmer 1 Yellow Light Food
MONO SLIMMERS (List C Foods)			
Fats, Oils, Spreads	≤ 240 mg per serving	Limit to 100 calories per meal	1 Mono Slimmer
Seeds, Nuts, Nut butters, Sauces, Hummus, Olives	≤240 mg per serving on label; 241–600 mg per serving	Limit nuts, seeds, olives to 100 calories Limit to 100 calories	1 Mono Slimmer 1 Yellow Light Food
FLUSHERS AND ANTI-BLOATERS (List D Foods)			
Non-Starchy Vegetables, Fruits, Non-starchy Tomato Sauce; fresh and canned/ processed	≤240 mg per serving 240–600 mg per serving	≤50 calories for vegetables and tomato sauce, ≤100 calorie permitted for fruit ≤ 100 calories for fruits canned in own juice only, no syrup Beans and vegetables must be rinsed	1 Flusher/ Anti-Bloater 1 Yellow Light Food
CONDIMENTS			
Freebies	≤20 mg per serving	≤10 calories	1 Freebie
	≤40 mg sodium per serving	≤20–25 calories	2 Freebies

Maintenance Food	Sodium Limit (2,300 mg a day)	Maintenance Slimmer Serving Qualifications	Count Each Serving As
CONDIMENTS *continued*			
Sauces, Dressings, Condiments, Snacks, Desserts	≤240 mg per serving on label	Allow one condiment daily with ≤240 mg sodium or several condiments that total 60 calories and 240 mg (see page 266–269)	1 Condiment
Beverages	≤140 mg/ per serving	Calorie-free beverages only *Limit diet soda (discouraged) and Crystal Light to one a day *Seltzer and calorie-free, sodium-free beverages with sugar-free sweetener (avoid if bloating occurs)	1 Beverage Slimmer
Convenience Slimmers: Entrees, sandwiches, prepared meats, soups, main dishes, meals	≤400 mg per serving	Limit entrees to one daily). Entrees (frozen/ prepared) ≤320 calories, ≤10 grams fat; ≤ 2 grams saturated fat; (ideally ≥5 grams protein, ≥3 grams fiber). If food exceeeds fat or calorie requirement, it is a Yellow Light Food.	Use calories as guide to count number of Slimmers (see page 281)
	400–600 mg sodium per serving	See qualifications in lists on page 254	Yellow Light Food

Carbohydrate Slimmers on the Maintenance Plan

As you no doubt witnessed during the ten days of the Jumpstart phase, whole grains help you feel satisfied. If you continue to choose bread products (breads, English muffins, pitas, wraps, and so on) and cereals from the Jumpstart Plan (List A in Appendix I), then there is no reason that all of your Carbohydrate Slimmer servings can't come from bread and cereal products. However, if you choose breads and cereals from the new list (List A in Appendix II), you'll have to limit these foods to two of your daily Carbohydrate Slimmers, since the sodium can accumulate quickly. You can get your remaining Carbohydrate Slimmers from rice, corn, sweet potatoes, steel-cut and old-fashioned oatmeal, quinoa and other grains, and any other non-bread or cereal option on List A. Do your best to choose breads with 150 milligrams of sodium or less, although many will have more. You'll

Nutrition Twins FAVORITE

Pepperidge Farm Whole Grain
100% Whole Wheat

find that lower-sodium whole-grain crackers, such as Wasa crackers, also fit into the Maintenance Plan.

The Yellow Light cereals either fall slightly short when it comes to fiber (1 to 2 grams below other Slimmers) or are slightly high in sugar (a gram or two more than the guidelines) or salt (100 milligrams more than other Slimmers). Some cereals on this list have up to 10 extra calories; we allow them to qualify as Yellow Light foods as long as they meet the other requirements.

RICE

Even in the Maintenance phase, you'll still have to avoid most rice mixes, as few have less than 240 milligrams of sodium per serving.

(Check out Goya Low Sodium Yellow Rice for a rare exception.) There's good news for sushi lovers, though. If you can't get brown rice sushi you can still have sushi on occasion. White rice contains no bloating sodium, so you can eat white rice and count it as a Yellow Light

> **Quaker Instant Oatmeal,** Lower Sugar Maple and Brown Sugar Flavor, contains over 100 milligrams more sodium than their Lower Sugar Apples & Cinnamon flavor (290 milligrams versus 170 milligrams).

food. Just be sure to have a Flusher with it, like leafy greens or carrots.

CORN, PEAS, POTATOES, WINTER SQUASH, AND BUTTERNUT SQUASH

You can eat any of these canned. Still aim for varieties without added salt (or sugar). Otherwise, be smart and rinse canned vegetables to lower the sodium content. Of course frozen is still a better option since salt isn't added and the nutrients are intact.

Protein Slimmers on the Maintenance Plan

As you've witnessed, Protein Slimmers take longer to digest than Carbohydrate Slimmers, thereby lengthening the energy boost of the Carbohydrate Slimmers and making you feel more satiated. You will find additions to the Protein Slimmers in List B in Appendix II. Several meats on the Protein Slimmers list are fairly high in calories despite being Slimmers. For these meats, smaller serving sizes will be listed.

We urge you to be as active as possible. If for some reason you are unable to meet the exercise recommendations in this plan, you will need to consume fewer servings of both Carbohydrate and Protein Slimmers, or ideally, limit the Red Light foods to one a week.

LEGUMES

This category includes split peas, lentils, and beans (excluding green or wax beans). If you were hesitant to eat beans in the Jumpstart phase due to fear of bloating, it's now time to test your level of tolerance. Start gradually, increasing the amount of beans you eat and the frequency. This will give your body a chance to adjust. Start by sprinkling just 2 tablespoons on your salad, in your pasta, or in your soup. Record the results in your Food Log. Continue to increase by 1 tablespoon every time you eat beans over the next two weeks until you reach one serving (½ cup). As you increase your intake, should you have any issues, try Beano. Continue to journal the results. If you have bean sensitivities, Beano may make you feel much better.

Fat-free refried beans and baked beans without pork (baked beans with pork is a Bloater) are higher in sodium than regular canned beans but are otherwise very healthy, so they're Yellow Light foods. These will be limited to ⅓-cup servings as noted in List B in Appendix II.

Avoiding Protein Overload

What happens when there's too much protein in your diet? Among other things, too much protein will actually cause you to gain body fat. A diet that is too high in protein exacerbates fatigue. Protein takes a long time to digest (about four to six hours versus the one-half to four hours that it takes to digest and burn up carbohydrates). Although protein's slower digestion can be a good thing (it promotes satiety when you combine the right amounts of the Carbohydrate Slimmers with the appropriate portions of the Protein Slimmers), too much protein creates problems. Eating a large quantity of protein at one sitting causes more blood to leave the brain and muscles and remain in your stomach (and intestine) for a longer period of time for digestion. As a result, there is less blood available to supply the muscles and brain with oxygen, causing sluggishness and decreased energy. This drop in energy, in turn, results in your being less active and burning fewer calories.

MEAT

When it comes to meat, continue to ban smoked varieties, and beware of the sodium in deli meats. Some of Oscar Mayer's and Louis Rich's meats have more than 600 milligrams per 2 ounces and can hit 700 or 800 milligrams per serving.

FISH

On the Maintenance Plan, you can eat canned fish that isn't labeled "low in sodium" or "no salt added"; however, you should still rinse it. With a few exceptions (those listed in Appendix II), steer clear of canned fish that is already seasoned—it will have far more than the 240-milligram sodium limit in 2 ounces. Although the fish that are highest in omega-3 fatty acids, such as salmon, herring, anchovies, oysters, sardines, whitefish, and mackerel, have many benefits, their portion size is slightly smaller (1½ ounces) because they are higher in calories than other fish.

> **Nutrition Twins FAVORITE**
>
> Bearitos Fat Free Green Chili Refried Beans. We stick to ⅓-cup servings to help keep the sodium at bay. They are delicious, so it's worth the Yellow Light food price tag for the day.

Weight-Saving SWAP Check out this swap: You can have 2 ounces of plain canned tuna for 240 milligrams sodium, or you can have 2 ounces of very-low-sodium canned tuna with a tablespoon of fat-free mayonnaise and a teaspoon of Hellmann's Dijonnaise for a total of 225 milligrams sodium—a 15-milligram sodium savings. Since the low-sodium canned tuna option falls below the 240-milligram sodium requirement for 2 ounces of canned fish, you don't even have to count those condiments toward your Condiment Slimmer allotment.

Mono Slimmers on the Maintenance Plan

As you've witnessed, Mono Slimmers add great flavor to food, and they take longer to digest than Carbohydrate Slimmers, making you feel more satiated. Now, you'll find that you can have salted nuts (and their butters) and olives. You will find the new additions to the Mono Slimmers in List C in Appendix III. (Several Mono Slimmers are fairly high in sodium, and they will be noted and counted as Yellow Light foods. Portions are still limited to keep calories in check.

OLIVES

The olives that are labeled Yellow Light foods count as your Yellow Light food for the day since the sodium content is greater than 240 milligrams. Instead of having them take the place of a Carbohydrate or Protein Slimmer, you can have them replace half your Mono Slimmer serving (since they have roughly half the calories of a Mono Slimmer [100 calories]).

 When you eat olives, select the chopped ones; the flavor gets dispersed throughout your meal, so they go further. The greener the olive oil, the more antioxidants. So go for extra-virgin green olives when you can.

SALTED NUTS AND SALTED NUT BUTTERS

Because each serving size is small, sticking to a serving keeps the sodium in check at 80 to 150 milligrams or less. For the best results, limit salted nuts, especially salted peanuts; they're smaller, so they have a larger surface area, which means there is more area that gets covered with salt. If you have more than one serving, count it as your Yellow Light food for the day. Don't worry—you'll easily adjust to the unsalted variety and your flatter stomach!

Avoid reduced-fat peanut butter. The calories are *no less* than the regular. The heart-healthy fat is replaced with sugar and/or carbohydrate filler. Plus the sodium is jacked up. A tablespoon of reduced-fat Jif peanut butter (125 milligrams sodium) has almost twice the sodium that regular peanut butter has (75 milligrams).

Flushers and Anti-Bloaters on the Maintenance Plan

By now you have witnessed the magical slimming power of fruits and vegetables. As you can see in Table 4 at the beginning of this chapter, you can include more canned varieties on the Maintenance Plan. Vegetables (including tomato sauce) with less than 240 milligrams of sodium and less than 50 calories per serving all fit your new plan; however, there's no excuse not to rinse salt off your canned veggies.

> **Nutrition Twins FAVORITE**
>
> PB2. We love this powdered peanut butter! We know it sounds bizarre, but we can pack this in a plastic bag without a sticky mess. Plus, it is super lightweight, and we can travel with it and just add a little water to make it into the real deal. Our favorite part? You get 4 tablespoons for 100 calories compared to just 1 tablespoon of regular peanut butter.

Just as in the Jumpstart phase, if your Green Light Flusher or Anti-Bloater is swimming in butter—you have to count that butter—it's a Red Light food. And if it's cooked in olive oil, remember to count it as a Mono Slimmer serving—calories can accumulate faster than you can blink. If you must get fruit canned in syrup, be sure it's "lite" syrup; have just ½ cup and count it as a Yellow Light food since Flushers and Anti-Bloaters should only contain naturally occurring sugars.

Think you are doing yourself a favor by drinking vegetable juice? Don't be fooled—a cup of regular V8 vegetable juice contains 480 milligrams of sodium, 20 percent of the day's allotment. A low-sodium V8 isn't great either; it still has 140 milligrams of sodium. If you want to drink vegetable juice, juice the veggies yourself. Better yet, drink water and eat your veggies—that way you get the flushing fiber and the slimming benefits of water, too.

Beverage Slimmers on the Maintenance Plan

During the Jumpstart phase, you were permitted to drink water, tea, and a daily coffee, and for optimal health these should still be your primary beverages. But on the Maintenance Plan, you can now consume other calorie-free beverages, as long as they have less than 140 milligrams of sodium. You must limit diet soda or diet drinks such as Crystal Light to one 12-ounce serving daily to keep the unnatural stuff like artificial sweeteners to a minimum. Besides, soda is bloating. If you were a soda drinker, you have seen this for yourself. However, now, after the Jumpstart Phase, you look and feel much leaner. Seltzer is a fantastic beverage but journal your response as many people get bloated from the carbonation.

Convenience Foods on the Maintenance Plan

In general, you'll use calories as your guide when counting servings of Convenience Slimmers. If a prepared convenience food has 100 calories or less, you can count that as either one of your Carbohydrate Slimmers or one of your Protein Slimmers, but usually you'll count it as half of each. That's because frozen entrées and other prepared meals usually have some carbs and some protein. If a Convenience Food has 101 to 150 calories, you'll count it as 1½ Slimmer servings. If it has 151 to 200 calories, it will count as 2 servings. From 201 to 250 calories? That's 2½ servings, and 251 to 310 calories is 3 servings. You get the idea. And you'll track 3 servings as 1.5 Protein Slimmers and 1.5 Carbohydrate Slimmers unless it is not a combination food. For instance, if you choose a 190-calorie prepared turkey patty as your Convenience food, turkey is obviously protein and therefore would count as two Protein Slimmer servings. Tracking convenience foods like this will ensure that you hold yourself accountable for all the food that you eat and that you continue to lose weight.

Frozen Entrees: In general, look for the healthiest frozen meals—many are listed in Appendix II. Don't see your favorite in the Appendix? It may still qualify if it meets the frozen entrée guidelines given in Table 4 at the beginning of this chapter.

CONVENIENCE SLIMMERS (NOT ENTRÉES)

The best "prepared" proteins have less than 1 gram of saturated fat. Remember, if it meets all Convenience Slimmer requirements in Table 4, except slightly falls outside of the range for one category, it's a Yellow Light food. But if a meat has more than 600 milligrams of sodium per 2 ounces, it's a Bloater and you'll count it as 1 Red Light food.

Building a Better Sandwich

Compare this healthy turkey sandwich to the Convenience Slimmers or a typical sub you might buy at a deli with a white roll and overstuffed portions of meat, which could top 800 calories!

Try this Turkey Sandwich made with:
- 2 slices of Pepperidge Farm 100% Whole Wheat Bread = 220 calories, 300 mg sodium, 6 g fiber, 8 g protein, 3 g fat, 40 g carbohydrates
- 2 ounces of honey roasted, thick sliced turkey breast = 60 calories, 500 mg sodium, 10 g protein, 2 carbs (Deli poultry with 480–600 mg sodium per 2-ounce serving counts as a Yellow Light Slimmer).
- Lettuce and tomato = negligible calories and fiber
- 1 teaspoon of mustard = 120 mg sodium
- Apple slices layered in sandwich = 94 calories, 2 mg sodium, 4.5 grams fiber, .05 protein, 25 g carbs
- 1 cup bell pepper slices = 18 calories, 1.6 g fiber, 4.3 g carbs **Total: 402 calories, 920 mg sodium, 4 g fat, 12 g fiber, 19 g protein, 70 g carbs** (2 Carbohydrate Slimmers, 1 Protein Slimmer, 2 Flushers, ½ Condiment Slimmer)

Try these swaps for even bigger savings:
- Choose 1 teaspoon Dijonnaise instead of mustard, and the sodium in your meal drops to 870 mg.
- Choose 2 ounces low-sodium turkey, and your meal drops to 680 mg sodium.
- Choose low-sodium turkey and Dijonnaise, and you'll be down to 630 mg sodium.
- Choose a teaspoon of cranberry sauce instead of Dijonnaise, and you're down to 560 mg sodium.

ENERGY BARS

For the most part, we don't recommend energy bars because many of them are nutritionally equal to candy bars; they're categorized as Red Light foods. Don't be fooled: just because many bars have added protein, vitamins, minerals, or even antioxidants, they are usually processed and refined. Although some bars are low in fat, others can have as much total fat and saturated fat as a Snickers bar.

However, we do realize that you may want a bar on occasion, so we have created guidelines to help you to find the best ones. First, eat bars only as a snack—not as a meal replacement—as they rarely provide the nutrients that you need from a meal, and they're likely to leave you hungry. Look for bars with less than 200 calories, no more than 1 gram of saturated fat, at least 3 grams of fiber, and no more than 12 grams of sugar. Look for bars that say "no added sugars"; their sugar content is all naturally occurring from fruit.

As with other Convenience Slimmers, use calories as your guide to count servings of energy bars. If a bar is made of nuts and fruits, then those nuts can count toward your Mono Slimmer servings. Remember, one of our favorite bars, a "Nutrition Twins Favorite," is actually a Carbohydrate Slimmer on the Jumpstart list (Gnu bar). It doesn't have protein, though, so you'd want to have it with a yogurt or low-fat string cheese or another Protein Slimmer to keep you feeling satisfied longer. (See recipe on page 199 for our Nutrition Twins Skinny & Quick Peanut Bars—they are a good "on-the-go" replacement for commercial bars.)

> Per FDA requirements, in order for a product to say "healthy" on the label it must be low in fat and saturated fat and contain limited amounts of cholesterol and sodium. If it's a single-item food, it must provide at least 10 percent of one or more of vitamins A or C, iron, calcium, protein, or fiber. The sodium content cannot exceed 360 mg per serving for individual foods and 480 mg per serving for meal-type products.

SOUPS

Soup servings are 1 cup. The list in Appendix II is just a sampling of soups considered "healthy." If you don't see your soup on the list in Table 4, your best bet is to make sure it meets the "healthy" guidelines (≤360 mg sodium; ≤3 grams of fat; ≤1 gram of saturated fat; must provide 10 percent Daily Value of vitamin A, vitamin C, iron, calcium, protein [less than or equal to 5 grams] and have 2.5 grams of fiber or more). Remember, try to get your soup with "no salt added," and you can always add extra flavor with spices. To follow the same guidelines as for other Convenience Slimmers, you'll need to look for those soups with less than 400 milligrams of sodium. Soups with 400 to 600 milligrams of sodium are Yellow Light foods. So, although some cans may say "healthy" on the label, they still only fall into the Yellow Light food category.

Want an easy way to add an Anti-Bloater to your soup? Dump a bag of frozen veggies (or two) into your canned soup when you heat it. Toss frozen green beans or spinach in minestrone; frozen carrots and onions in chicken noodle soup; a frozen vegetable medley in Manhattan clam chowder; and frozen cauliflower and peppers into tomato soup. And why limit this to soups? Dump frozen veggies in any pasta, casserole, omelet, and more!

Studies have shown that when you eat soup as a first course, especially vegetable soups, you'll eat about 100 fewer calories in that meal. Also, eating chicken and rice soup reduced calorie intake of subsequent meals more effectively than eating the ingredients (chicken and rice) separately followed by a glass of water. Although we'd love you to make your own delicious, low-sodium soup all of the time (see page 221 for a simple recipe), we are realistic. And luckily, although many canned soups are drowning in sodium, companies like Progresso and Campbell's now offer lower-sodium options that have 480 milligrams of sodium per serving, about half the 870 milligrams of sodium found in their other soups. These soups help you fill up, eat less of other foods, and keep you from swelling like there's no tomorrow. Still, like other Convenience foods that have between 400 and 600 milligrams of sodium, you'll have to count them as Yellow Light foods. You'll see these soups and some others that fit the bill in Appendix II.

 If you must use a butter-like spread, avoid the artery-clogging saturated fat found in butter and choose a spread like I Can't Believe It's Not Butter!, Promise, or Country Crock soft spreads, which are a better nutritional option than butter because they are lower in fat, saturated fat (70–80% less), and cholesterol, and contain 0 grams trans fat per serving. They're made with a blend of nutritious vegetable oils such as canola, soybean, and olive oil.

Condiments and Miscellaneous Foods on the Maintenance Plan

In addition to the Freebies you were allotted in the Jumpstart phase, you can have one condiment with less than 60 calories per serving and less than 240 milligrams of sodium. You could also choose to have two half-serving condiments that have a combined total 60 calories and up to 240 milligrams of sodium. In order to meet these guidelines, some condiment serving sizes will need to be made smaller (such as Kraft Mayonnaise with Olive Oil, or Marie's Raspberry Vinaigrette). We have done the work for you by cutting serving sizes of many of the condiments in Appendix II, so they equal half servings (30 calories and 120-milligrams of sodium). This way you can mix and match and choose two a day. Some foods must count as your full Condiment serving because their calories and/or sodium fall above the 30 calories and 120-milligram sodium range, but cutting the portion in half isn't realistic (see Appendix II List E).

If you refuse to give up your mayo, here's an option—Kraft Mayonnaise with Olive Oil. It has half the fat and calories of regular mayo. A tablespoon has 45 calories, 4 grams of fat, 95 milligrams of sodium, and no trans or saturated fat. Not too bad. You can have 2 teaspoons (30 calories, 62 milligrams sodium) and use only one-half of your daily Slimmer Condiment serving.

Now that you know more about the foods you can enjoy on the Maintenance Plan, the next chapter gives you two weeks of Maintenance Plan menus to make meal planning that much easier.

Chapter 7

Two Weeks of Maintenance Plan Menus

By successfully completing the Jumpstart Plan, you showed tremendous willpower, which should be paying off with a leaner, bloat-free body and increased energy levels. In this chapter you'll find two weeks of menus for women and men. Once you familiarize yourself with the foods that will maintain your weight loss, you'll be able to mix and match your own meals in no time. Be sure to check out the Red Light foods in chapter 8, too. While the Maintenance Plan permits these foods in *small* quantities, you need to recognize the Red Light foods in your daily life and understand how detrimental they are to your fitness goals and the new slimmer you.

Maintenance Day 1 Women

Breakfast

½ Sara Lee Healthy Whole Wheat Cinnamon Raisin Bagel (1½ Carb Slimmers)

¾ cup nonfat ricotta cheese, spread on your bagel with a sprinkle of cinnamon
(1½ Protein Slimmers)

½ large banana (1 Flusher/Anti-Bloater)

2 cups green tea (2 Beverage Slimmers)

Lunch

3 ounces grilled or baked chicken breast (1½ Protein Slimmers) with Mrs. Dash
Mesquite Grille 10-Minute Marinade (2 Freebies)

4½-ounce baked potato, the size of your fist, or ½ large baked potato
(1½ Carb Slimmers)

1½ teaspoons bacon bits (½ Condiment)

2 tablespoons fat-free sour cream (2 Freebies)

1 cup steamed broccoli spritzed with lemon (2 Flushers/Anti-Bloaters)

1 cup water, 1 cup tea (2 Beverage Slimmers)

Mid-Afternoon Snack

30 unsalted pistachios (1 Mono Slimmer)

1 orange (1 Flusher/Anti-Bloater)

1 cup water (1 Beverage Slimmer)

Dinner

Mixed Greens Salad made with:

2 cups mixed greens

½ cup sliced tomatoes

¼ cup shredded carrots

¼ cup sliced zucchini (3 Flushers/Anti-Bloaters)

1 tablespoon Annies Naturals Lite Honey Mustard Vinaigrette (½ Condiment)

Peppery Tuna Grill *(See recipe page 189)* (2 Protein Slimmers, 1½ Flushers/ Anti-Bloaters)

½ serving Mushroom Barley Risotto *(See recipe page 216)*
(1 Carb Slimmer, ½ Mono Slimmer, ½ Flusher/Anti-Bloater)

2 cups water (2 Beverage Slimmers)

After-Dinner Snack *(at least an hour before bed)* •••••••••••••••••••••••••••••••••

Skinny Cow Ice Cream Cone (1 Red Light Food)

2 cups green tea (2 Beverage Slimmers)

> DAILY TOTAL: Calories 1,385, Fat 30 grams, Saturated Fat 7 grams, Carbohydrates 163 grams, Protein 123 grams, Fiber 27 grams, Sodium 1,537 milligrams
> 4 Carb Slimmers, 5 Protein Slimmers, 1½ Mono Slimmers, 9 Flushers/Anti-Bloaters, 9 Beverage Slimmers, 1 Red Light Food, 1 Condiment, 4 Freebies

Maintenance Day 1 Men

Lunch: Add 3 ounces grilled chicken breast and have a larger baked potato, about 6 ounces or the size of your fist. Also add an additional ½ cup broccoli.

> DAILY TOTAL: Calories 1,600, Carbohydrates 190 grams, Protein 145 grams, Total Fat 32 grams, Saturated Fat 8 grams, Fiber 32 grams, Sodium 1,607 milligrams
> 5 Carb Slimmers, 6½ Protein Slimmers, 1½ Mono Slimmers, 9 Flushers/Anti-Bloaters, 9 Beverage Slimmers, 1 Red Light Food, 1 Condiment, 4 Freebies

Maintenance Day 2 Women

Breakfast ••

Quaker Instant Oatmeal Lower Sugar Apple and Cinnamon (1 Carb Slimmer)

½ sliced apple, added to oatmeal (½ Flusher/Anti-Bloater)

6 ounces Stonyfield Nonfat Plain Yogurt (1 Protein Slimmer) *(can mix into oatmeal, or sprinkle with cinnamon and add the apple to it)*

2 cups water, 1 cup green tea (3 Beverage Slimmers)

Lunch

Chicken Sandwich made with:

½ cup Perdue Shortcuts Honey Flavored Carved Chicken Breast
   (1 Yellow Light Food)

2 slices Pepperidge Farm 100% Whole Grain Whole Wheat (2 Carb Slimmers)

Slice tomato and 2 inner leaves of lettuce (¼ Flusher/Anti-Bloater)

1 teaspoon Dijonnaise (½ Condiment)

1 Steamfresh Singles Baby Brussels Sprouts (2 Flushers/Anti-Bloaters)

1 cup cubed cantaloupe (1 Flusher/Anti-Bloater)

2 cups water (2 Beverage Slimmers)

Snack

1 Gnu Bar (1 Carb Slimmer)

1 Trader Joe's Light Organic String Cheese (1 Protein Slimmer)

½ apple (½ Flusher/Anti-Bloater)

2 cups tea (2 Beverage Slimmers)

Dinner

Peruvian Ceviche with Potatoes, Halibut, and Mango *(See recipe page 190)*
(1 Carb Slimmer, 1 Protein Slimmer) **served on:**

1 ounce baked tortilla chips (1 Red Light Food)

1½ cups steamed mixed vegetables sprinkled with lemon juice
   (3 Flushers/Anti-Bloaters) and 1 tablespoon slivered almonds (½ Mono Slimmer)

1 cup water, 1 cup green tea (2 Beverage Slimmers)

After-Dinner Snack *(at least an hour before bed)*

2 Ryvita Light Rye Crisp Bread crackers (1 Carb Slimmer)

1 The Laughing Cow, Mini Babybel, Light Original Cheese (1 Protein Slimmer)

1 cup green tea (1 Beverage Slimmer)

DAILY TOTAL: Calories 1,463, Carbohydrates 253 grams, Fat 27 grams, Saturated Fat 6 grams, Protein 76 grams, Fiber 45 grams, Sodium 1,982 milligrams
5 Carb Slimmers *(extra Carb instead of 1 Red Light option)*, 5 Protein Slimmers, ½ Mono Slimmer, ½ Condiment, 7¼ Flushers/Anti-Bloaters, 10 Beverage Slimmers, 1 Yellow Light Food, 1 Red Light Food

Maintenance Day 2 Men

Dinner: Add an extra serving of Peruvian Ceviche with Potatoes, Halibut, and Mango. **After-Dinner Snack:** Add ½ Laughing Cow Mini Babybel Light Original Cheese.

DAILY TOTAL: Calories 1,646, Carbohydrates 273 grams, Protein 96 grams, Total Fat 29 grams, Saturated Fat 6 grams, Fiber 47 grams, Sodium 2,236 milligrams
6 Carb Slimmers *(extra Carb instead of 1 Red Light Food)*, 6½ Protein Slimmers, ½ Mono Slimmer, ½ Condiment, 7¼ Flushers/Anti-Bloaters, 10 Beverage Slimmers, 1 Yellow Light Food, 1 Red Light Food

Maintenance Day 3 Women

Breakfast

Crunchy Yogurt Parfait made with:

6 ounces Yoplait Light Strawberry Yogurt (1 Protein Slimmer)

1 cup Kashi Go Lean (1½ Carb Slimmers)

½ banana (1 Flusher/Anti-Bloater)

2 sliced strawberries (¼ Flusher/Anti-Bloater)

1 teaspoon sunflower seeds (⅙ Mono Slimmer)

To Make: In a glass, layer the following: ¼ cup yogurt, ¼ cup cereal, strawberries, and sliced bananas. Top with sunflower seeds. Layer again with remaining ingredients.

1 cup water, 2 cups green tea (3 Beverage Slimmers)

Lunch

Spinach, Pear, and Salmon Salad with Vinaigrette Dressing made with:

2 cups spinach (2 Flushers/Anti-Bloaters)

½ cup broccoli florets (½ Flusher/Anti-Bloater)

½ cup shredded carrots (½ Flusher/Anti-Bloater)

½ cup tomatoes (½ Flusher/Anti-Bloater)

2 ounces canned or fresh salmon (1¼ Protein Slimmers)

2 tablespoons Vinaigrette Salad Dressing *(See recipe page 224)* (3 Freebies)

1 pear, sliced (1 Flusher/Anti-Bloater)

1 whole-grain roll (1 Carb Slimmer)

10 sprays I Can't Believe It's Not Butter! spray (1 Freebie)

2 cups water (2 Beverage Slimmers)

Mid-Afternoon Snack

Amy's Bistro Burger (1 Protein Slimmer) **on a bed of:**

1 cup chopped Romaine lettuce (1 Flusher/Anti-Bloater)

1 cup baby carrots (1 Flusher/Anti-Bloater)

2 tablespoons Marie's Raspberry Vinaigrette for dipping (½ Condiment)

1 cup green tea (1 Beverage Slimmer)

Dinner

Blazing Glory Raspberry Chicken Breasts
(See recipe page 182) (2 Protein Slimmers)

½ cup black beans *(rinsed, drained)* (1 Carb Slimmer) seasoned with pepper,
    garlic, and fresh herbs, to taste

2 cups mixed greens and ½ cup chopped tomato
(2½ Flushers/Anti-Bloaters) **with:**

1½ teaspoons olive oil (½ Mono Slimmer)

Splash balsamic vinegar (Unlimited)

1 cup water, 1 cup green tea (2 Beverage Slimmers)

After-Dinner Snack *(at least an hour before bed)* ··

5 ounces red wine (1 Red Light Food)

3 cups salted popcorn (1 Red Light Food)

> DAILY TOTAL: Calories 1,450, Fat 22 grams, Saturated Fat 3 grams, Carbohydrates 227 grams, Protein 78 grams, Fiber 45 grams, Sodium 2,024 milligrams
> 3½ Carb Slimmers, 5¼ Protein Slimmers, 9¼ Flushers/Anti-Bloaters, ¾ Mono Slimmer, 8 Beverage Slimmers, 2 Red Light Foods, ½ Condiment, 4 Freebies

Maintenance Day 3 Men

Add 1 cup Kashi Go Lean to breakfast. Add 2 ounces of salmon at lunch and ½ Sargento Light String Cheese

> DAILY TOTAL: Calories 1,619, Carbohydrates 239 grams, Protein 95 grams, Total Fat 29 grams, Saturated Fat 5 grams, Fiber 45 grams, Sodium 2,300 milligrams
> 5 Carb Slimmers, 6½ Protein Slimmers, 9¼ Flushers/Anti-Bloaters, ¾ Mono Slimmer, 8 Beverage Slimmers, 2 Red Light Foods, ½ Condiment, 4 Freebies

Maintenance Day 4 Women

Breakfast ··

2 slices Cinnamon Orange French Toast *(See recipe page 205)*
  (2 Carb Slimmers, 1½ Protein Slimmers)

5 egg whites, scrambled in cooking spray (1¼ Protein Slimmers)

1 cup water, 2 cups green tea (3 Beverage Slimmers)

Lunch ···

Turkey Apple Sandwich made with:

2 slices Pepperidge Farm Whole Grain 100% Whole Wheat Bread (2 Carb Slimmers)

1 tablespoon fat-free mayonnaise (½ Condiment)

½ tablespoon Catalina dressing (½ Condiment)

3 ounces sliced Deli Fresh Shaved Smoked Turkey Breast (2 Red Light Foods)

½ apple *(cut into slices on sandwich)* (½ Flusher/Anti-Bloater)

1 cup baby carrots (1 Flusher/Anti-Bloater)

1 cup cantaloupe, cubed (1 Flusher/Anti-Bloater)

2 cups water (2 Beverage Slimmers)

Mid-Afternoon Snack

Skinny & Quick Peanut Bars *(See recipe page 199)* (1 Mono Slimmer, ¼ Protein Slimmer)

2 cups green tea (2 Beverage Slimmers)

Dinner

Asian Steak with Grapes *(See recipe page 179)* (2 Protein Slimmers, ¾ Flusher/
   Anti-Bloater)

1 cup steamed broccoli with lemon or butter spray (2 Flushers/Anti-Bloaters)

½ cup white rice (1 Yellow Light Food)

1 cup water, 1 cup green tea (2 Beverage Slimmers)

After-Dinner Snack *(at least an hour before bed)*

½ cup canned Libby's Pumpkin sprinkled with cinnamon and Splenda
   (or 1 teaspoon sugar) (1 Flusher/Anti-Bloater) on top of:

1 ounce Redi-Whip Fat Free whipped topping (2 Freebies)

1 cup green tea (1 Beverage Slimmer)

> DAILY TOTAL: Calories 1,411, Carbohydrates 199 grams, Protein 85 grams, Total Fat 35 grams, Saturated Fat 7 grams, Fiber 26 grams, Sodium 1,882 milligrams
> 4 Carb Slimmers, 5¼ Protein Slimmers, 1 Mono Slimmer, 6¼ Anti-Bloaters/Flushers, 2 Condiments, 10 Beverage Slimmers, 1 Yellow Light Food, 2 Red Light Foods, 2 Freebies

Maintenance Day 4 Men

Add ½ cup of brown rice at dinner and another ¾ serving of Asian Steak with Grapes.

> DAILY TOTAL: Calories 1,609, Carbohydrates 232 grams, Protein 90 grams, Total Fat 43 grams, Saturated Fat 9 grams, Dietary Fiber 28 grams, Sodium 2,124 milligrams
> 5 Carb Slimmers, 6¾ Protein Slimmers, 1 Mono Slimmer, 6¾ Anti-Bloaters/Flushers, 2 Condiments, 10 Beverage Slimmers, 1 Yellow Light Food, 2 Red Light Foods, 2 Freebies

Maintenance Day 5 Women

Breakfast

¾ cup pineapple, canned in own juice (1 Flusher/Anti-Bloater) mixed with:

½ cup low-fat cottage cheese (1 Protein Slimmer)

½ Pepperidge Farm Whole Grain 100% Whole Wheat English muffin
   (¾ Carb Slimmer)

1 cup water, 1 cup green tea (2 Beverage Slimmers)

Lunch

2 servings of Pesto Deviled Eggs *(See recipe page 191)* (2 Protein Slimmers)

Strawberry Fields salad with:

2 cups spinach (2 Flushers/Anti-Bloaters)

½ cup each tomato, squash, pepper, carrots (2 Flushers/Anti-Bloaters)

½ cup sliced strawberries (1 Flusher/Anti-Bloater)

2 tablespoons slivered pecans (1 Mono Slimmer)

2 Ryvita Sesame Rye Crispbread broken up in salad (1 Carb Slimmer)

2 cups water (2 Beverage Slimmers)

Mid-Afternoon Snack

Newman's Own Natural 100-Calorie Pack Mini Bag microwave popcorn
   (1 Carb Slimmer) sprinkled with 1 tablespoon grated Parmesan (½ Condiment)

1 low-fat string cheese (1 Protein Slimmer)

2 cups tea (2 Beverage Slimmers)

Dinner

Zucchini Lasagna *(See recipe page 198)* (1 Carb Slimmer, 1 Protein Slimmer,
   ½ Flusher/Anti-Bloater)

1 whole grain dinner roll, spread with roasted garlic and butter spray
   (1 Carb Slimmer)

1 cup steamed carrots, cauliflower, and snow peas (2 Flushers/Anti-Bloaters)

1 cup water, 1 cup tea (2 Beverage Slimmers)

After-Dinner Snack *(at least an hour before bed)* ···

Skinny Cow Vanilla Fudge pop (1 Red Light Food)

2 cups green tea (2 Beverage Slimmers)

> DAILY TOTAL: Calories 1,363, Carbohydrates 184 grams, Protein 81 grams, Total Fat 40 grams,
> Saturated Fat 10 grams, Fiber 29 grams, Sodium 1,690 milligrams
> 4¾ Carb Slimmers, 5 Protein Slimmers, 8½ Anti-Bloaters/Flushers, 1 Mono Slimmer,
> ½ Condiment, 10 Beverage Slimmers, 1 Red Light Food

Maintenance Day 5 Men

At breakfast, add another quarter-cup of cottage cheese. At dinner, add another
serving of lasagna, totaling 2 servings.

> DAILY TOTAL: Calories 1,612, Carbohydrates 211 grams, Protein 106 grams, Total Fat 45
> grams, Saturated Fat 13 grams, Fiber 32 grams, Sodium 2,160 milligrams
> 5¾ Carb Slimmers, 6½ Protein Slimmers, 9 Flushers/Anti-Bloaters, 1 Mono Slimmer,
> ½ Condiment, 10 Beverage Slimmers, 1 Red Light Food

Maintenance Day 6 Women

Breakfast ··

2 4-inch pancakes made from Quaker Oatmeal Pancake mix; Use heart-healthy
directions (2 Carb Slimmers, ¼ Protein Slimmer)

¼ cup blueberries *(add into pancake mix)* (½ Flusher/Anti-Bloater)

4 tablespoons sugar-free syrup (½ Condiment)

2 ounces Oscar Mayer Canadian bacon (1 Yellow Light Food)

1 cup water, 2 cups tea (3 Beverage Slimmers)

Lunch ···

Peanut Butter Banana Roll-Up *(See recipe page 200)* made with:

1 medium banana (1 Flusher/Anti-Bloater)

3 tablespoons Smucker's All Natural Peanut Butter, or other all-natural brand
(1 Mono Slimmer)

1 slice Alvarado Street Bakery No Salt! Sprouted Multi-Grain Bread
(or other low-sodium whole-wheat bread) (1 Carb Slimmer)

1 tablespoon sugar-free jelly (1 Freebie)

1 cup each cucumber and carrot strips (2 Flushers/Anti-Bloaters)

½ cup low-fat cottage cheese (1 Protein Slimmer)

2 cups water (2 Beverage Slimmers)

Mid-Afternoon Snack

1 hard-boiled egg (1 Protein Slimmer)

½ cup strawberries (½ Flusher/Anti-Bloater)

6 ounces Yoplait Light Strawberry flavor yogurt (1 Protein Slimmer)

1 cup green tea (1 Beverage Slimmer)

Dinner

2 servings Ginger Shrimp with Gai Lan *(See recipe page 185)*
(2 Protein Slimmers, ⅓ Mono Slimmer)

2 cups bok choy and greens (2 Flushers/Anti-Bloaters) sautéed with:

2 tablespoons low-sodium chicken or veggie broth (1 Freebie)

½ cup brown rice (1 Carb Slimmer)

1 cup water, 1 cup tea (2 Beverage Slimmers)

After-Dinner Snack (at least one hour before bed)

2 Fat Free Fig Newtons (1 Red Light Food)

1 cup green tea (1 Beverage Slimmer)

DAILY TOTAL: Calories 1,425, Carbohydrates 220 grams, Protein 80 grams, Total Fat 31 grams, Saturated Fat 5.5 grams, Fiber 27 grams, Sodium 1,919 milligrams
4 Carb Slimmers, 5 Protein Slimmers, 1⅓ Mono Slimmers, 6 Flushers/Anti-Bloaters, 9 Beverage Slimmers, 1 Yellow Light Food, 1 Red Light Food, 2 Freebies, ½ Condiment

Maintenance Day 6 Men

Add another slice of bread at lunch and another ¼ cup of cottage cheese. Add
another hard-boiled egg for an afternoon snack. Add ½ cup bok choy sautéed
in 2 tablespoons low-sodium chicken or veggie broth.

DAILY TOTAL: Calories 1,625, Carbohydrates 236 grams, Total Fat 39 grams, Saturated Fat 8
grams, Protein 95 grams, Dietary Fiber 32 grams, Sodium 2,231 milligrams
5 Carb Slimmers, 6½ Protein Slimmers, 1⅓ Mono Slimmers, 7 Flushers/Anti-Bloaters,
9 Beverage Slimmers, 1 Yellow Light Food, 1 Red Light Food, 3 Freebies, ½ Condiment

Maintenance Day 7 Women

Breakfast

1 cup Kashi Go Lean (1½ Carb Slimmers)

1 cup skim milk (1 Protein Slimmer)

4 chopped apricots (1 Flusher/Anti-Bloater)

2 cups green tea (2 Beverage Slimmers)

Lunch

2 slices Pepperidge Farm Whole Grain 100% Whole Wheat Bread
  (2 Carb Slimmers)

4 ounces Perdue Sliced Turkey Breast (2 Protein Slimmers)

2 leaves of lettuce, 2 slices of tomato (½ Flusher/Anti-Bloater)

2 teaspoons mustard (½ Condiment)

1 cup celery stalks (1 Flusher/Anti-Bloater)

1 cup grape tomatoes (1 Flusher/Anti-Bloater)

1 cup green tea, 1 cup water (2 Beverage Slimmers)

Mid-Afternoon Snack

1 apple (1 Flusher/Anti-Bloater)

3 teaspoons Smucker's All Natural Peanut Butter (1 Mono Slimmer)

2 cups water (2 Beverage Slimmers)

READER/CUSTOMER CARE SURVEY

HEFG

We care about your opinions! Please take a moment to fill out our online Reader Survey at **http://survey.hcibooks.com**.

As a **"THANK YOU"** you will receive a **VALUABLE INSTANT COUPON** towards future book purchases

as well as a **SPECIAL GIFT** available only online! Or, you may mail this card back to us.

(PLEASE PRINT IN ALL CAPS)

First Name		MI.		Last Name	
Address					City
State		Zip		Email	

1. Gender
- ❏ Female
- ❏ Male

2. Age
- ❏ 8 or younger
- ❏ 9-12
- ❏ 13-16
- ❏ 17-20
- ❏ 21-30
- ❏ 31+

3. Did you receive this book as a gift?
- ❏ Yes
- ❏ No

4. Annual Household Income
- ❏ under $25,000
- ❏ $25,000 - $34,999
- ❏ $35,000 - $49,999
- ❏ $50,000 - $74,999
- ❏ over $75,000

5. What are the ages of the children living in your house?
- ❏ 0 - 14
- ❏ 15+

6. Marital Status
- ❏ Single
- ❏ Married
- ❏ Divorced
- ❏ Widowed

7. How did you find out about the book?
(please choose one)
- ❏ Recommendation
- ❏ Store Display
- ❏ Online
- ❏ Catalog/Mailing
- ❏ Interview/Review

8. Where do you usually buy books?
(please choose one)
- ❏ Bookstore
- ❏ Online
- ❏ Book Club/Mail Order
- ❏ Price Club (Sam's Club, Costco's, etc.)
- ❏ Retail Store (Target, Wal-Mart, etc.)

9. What subject do you enjoy reading about the most?
(please choose one)
- ❏ Parenting/Family
- ❏ Relationships
- ❏ Recovery/Addictions
- ❏ Health/Nutrition
- ❏ Christianity
- ❏ Spirituality/Inspiration
- ❏ Business Self-help
- ❏ Women's Issues
- ❏ Sports

10. What attracts you most to a book?
(please choose one)
- ❏ Title
- ❏ Cover Design
- ❏ Author
- ❏ Content

TAPE IN MIDDLE; DO NOT STAPLE

BUSINESS REPLY MAIL
FIRST-CLASS MAIL PERMIT NO 45 DEERFIELD BEACH, FL

POSTAGE WILL BE PAID BY ADDRESSEE

Health Communications, Inc.
3201 SW 15th Street
Deerfield Beach FL 33442-9875

FOLD HERE

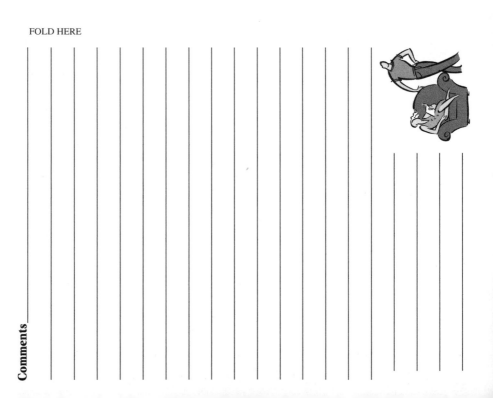

Comments

Dinner

2 ounces Perdue Fit & Easy Boneless, Skinless Chicken Breast (1 Protein Slimmer)

1 tablespoon KC Masterpiece BBQ Sauce (½ Condiment)

2 cups steamed broccoli and cauliflower (2 Flushers/Anti-Bloaters)

¼ cup wild rice (½ Carb Slimmer)

2 cups water (2 Beverage Slimmers)

After-Dinner Snack *(at least an hour before bed)*

8 Hershey's Kisses (2 Red Light Foods)

1 cup skim milk (1 Protein Slimmer)

1 cup green tea (1 Beverage Slimmer)

> DAILY TOTAL: Calories 1,420, Carbohydrates 169 grams, Protein 118 grams, Total Fat 30 grams, Saturated Fat 3 grams, Fiber 39 grams, Sodium 2,114 milligrams
> 4 Carb Slimmers, 5 Protein Slimmers, 6½ Anti-Bloaters/Flushers, 1 Mono Slimmer, 1 Condiment, 2 Red Light Foods, 9 Beverage Slimmers

Maintenance Day 7 Men

At dinner add another 3 ounces of chicken and another ½ cup of wild rice.

> DAILY TOTAL: Calories 1,587, Carbohydrates 186 grams, Total Fat 31 grams, Saturated Fat 4 grams, Protein 138 grams, Fiber 42 grams, Sodium 2,150 milligrams
> 5 Carb Slimmers, 6½ Protein Slimmers, 6½ Flushers/Anti-Bloaters, 1 Mono Slimmer, 1 Condiment, 2 Red Light Foods, 9 Beverage Slimmers

Maintenance Day 8 Women

Breakfast

Pepperidge Farm Whole Grain 100% Whole Wheat Mini Bagel
(1½ Carb Slimmers)

10 sprays I Can't Believe It's Not Butter! spray (1 Freebie)

Scrambled egg white omelet *(4 egg whites)* **cooked in cooking spray**
(1 Protein Slimmer) **with:**

½ ounce low-fat cheddar (½ Protein Slimmer)

½ cup of each—spinach, sliced mushrooms, sliced onions (1½ Flushers/Anti-Bloaters)

1 cup water, 1 cup green tea (2 Beverage Slimmers)

Lunch

Spaghetti and Turkey Tomato Sauce with vegetables:

1 cup whole-wheat pasta, cooked (2 Carb Slimmers)

3 ounces ground turkey breast *(sauté with onions and garlic in cooking spray)*
(1½ Protein Slimmers)

1¼ cups Walnut Acres Low Sodium Tomato and Basil Pasta Sauce
(2½ Flushers/Anti-Bloaters)

1 cup steamed broccoli *(mixed into turkey and pasta sauce)* (2 Flushers/Anti-Bloaters)

1 tablespoon grated Parmesan cheese *(sprinkle on top)* (½ Condiment)

1 cup water, 1 cup tea (2 Beverage Slimmers)

Mid-Afternoon Snack

30 pistachios (1 Mono Slimmer)

4 Sunsweet Ones Dried Plums (1 Flusher/Anti-Bloater)

1 cup tea (1 Beverage Slimmer)

Dinner

Chopped Salad (4 Flushers/Anti-Bloaters) **made with:**

2 cups chopped Romaine lettuce (2 Flushers/Anti-Bloaters)

½ cup chopped asparagus and green beans (½ Flusher/Anti-Bloater)

½ cup chopped tomato and carrots (½ Flusher/Anti-Bloater)

1 ounce nonfat mozzarella cheese shredded (1 Protein Slimmer)

10 sprays Wishbone Salad Spritzers Red Wine Mist or Raspberry Bliss
(½ Condiment)

Thai Pumpkin Soup *(See recipe page 222)* (1 Carb Slimmer, 1 Protein Slimmer,
⅓ Mono Slimmer)

1 Ryvita Fruit Crunch Crispbread (½ Carb Slimmer)

2 cups water, 1 cup tea (3 Beverage Slimmers)

After-Dinner Snack *(at least an hour before bed)* ∙∙∙∙∙∙∙∙∙∙∙∙∙∙∙∙∙∙∙∙∙∙∙∙∙∙∙∙∙∙∙∙∙

1 Skinny Cow Low-Fat Ice Cream Sandwich (1 Red Light Food)

1 cup tea (1 Beverage Slimmer)

> DAILY TOTAL: Calories 1,369, Carbohydrates 209 grams, Total Fat 28 grams, Saturated Fat 6 grams, Protein 95 grams, Fiber 38 grams, Sodium 1,479 milligrams
> 5 Carb Slimmers *(instead of 1 Red Light Food)*, 5 Protein Slimmers, 1⅓ Mono Slimmers, 11 Flushers/Anti-Bloaters, 1 Condiment, 9 Beverage Slimmers, 1 Red Light Food

Maintenance Day 8 Men

At lunch add another ½ cup of whole-wheat pasta and another 3 ounces of ground turkey breast.

> DAILY TOTAL: Calories 1,547, Carbohydrates 228 grams, Protein 119 grams, Total Fat 29 grams, Saturated Fat 6 grams, Fiber 40 grams, Sodium 1,542 milligrams
> 6 Carb Slimmers *(instead of 1 Red Light Food)*, 6½ Protein Slimmers, 1⅓ Mono Slimmers, 11 Flushers/Anti-Bloaters, 1 Condiment, 9 Beverage Slimmers, 1 Red Light Food

Maintenance Day 9 Women

Breakfast ∙∙

2 slices Weight Watchers Whole Wheat Bread *(or other reduced calorie, whole- wheat, high-fiber bread)* (1 Carb Slimmer)

½ cup Frigo nonfat ricotta cheese (1 Protein Slimmer)

¾ cup crushed pineapple, drained (1 Flusher/Anti-Bloater)

1 packet Carnation Sugar Free, Fat-Free Hot Chocolate (1 Condiment)

2 cups green tea (2 Beverage Slimmers)

Lunch ∙∙

Basil and Sundried Tomato Tuna on bed of greens:

3 ounces Creamy Sun-Dried Tomato Tuna *(See recipe page 210)* (1½ Protein Slimmers, ½ Mono Slimmer, 1 Flusher/Anti-Bloater)

2 cups mixed greens (2 Flushers/Anti-Bloaters)

2 cups sliced cucumber (2 Flushers/Anti-Bloaters)

2 Ryvita Crispbreads (1 Carb Slimmer), with cheese spread on top:

1 Laughing Cow Light Original Mini Babybel Cheese (1 Protein Slimmer)

1 apple (1 Flusher/Anti-Bloater)

1 cup nonfat pudding (1 Red Light Food)

1 cup tea, 1 cup water (2 Beverage Slimmers)

Snack

1 Trader Joe's Organic 100% Whole Wheat Pita (1 Carb Slimmer)

2½ tablespoons hummus (²/₃ Mono Slimmer)

1 cup baby carrots (1 Flusher/Anti-Bloater)

1 cup tea (1 Beverage Slimmer)

Dinner

Shrimp or Tofu Stir-Fry:

3 ounces firm tofu *(or shrimp)* (1½ Protein Slimmers)

1 clove of garlic (Unlimited)

½ teaspoon ginger (Unlimited)

⅛ teaspoon red pepper flakes (Unlimited)

Cooking spray (1 Freebie)

To Make: Stir-fry the garlic, ginger, and red pepper flakes in cooking spray, (1 Freebie) then add the vegetables and protein

½ cup each snow peas, carrots, broccoli, bell peppers (2 Flushers/Anti-Bloaters)

1 teaspoon lemon juice, for flavor (Unlimited)

½ cup brown rice (1 Carb Slimmer)

2 cups water (2 Beverage Slimmers)

After-Dinner Snack *(at least an hour before bed)*

2 Hershey's Miniatures (1 Red Light Food)

1 cup tea (1 Beverage Slimmer)

DAILY TOTAL: Calories 1,339, Carbohydrates 182 grams, Total Fat 37 grams, Saturated Fat 12 grams, Protein 80 grams, Fiber 33 grams, Sodium 1,472 milligrams
4 Carb Slimmers, 5 Protein Slimmers, 1⅓ Mono Slimmers, 10 Flushers/Anti-Bloaters, 8 Beverage Slimmers, 2 Red Light Foods, 1 Condiment, 1 Freebie

Maintenance Day 9 Men

At dinner, add ½ cup of rice and 3 ounces of firm tofu or shrimp.

DAILY TOTAL: Calories 1,587, Carbohydrates 215 grams, Protein 95 grams, Total Fat 45 grams, Saturated Fat 13 grams, Fiber 35 grams, Sodium 1,494 milligrams
5 Carb Slimmers, 6½ Protein Slimmers, 1⅓ Mono Slimmers, 10 Flushers/Anti-Bloaters, 8 Beverage Slimmers, 2 Red Light Foods, 1 Condiment, 1 Freebie

Maintenance Day 10 Women

Breakfast

1 serving *(½ cup raw)* Quaker Old Fashioned Oats (1½ Carb Slimmers)

½ cup Egg Beaters (1 Protein Slimmer) sautéed with:

1 teaspoon olive oil (⅓ Mono Slimmer)

¼ cup each onions, mushrooms, peppers, and spinach (1 Flusher/Anti-Bloater)

2 cups green tea (2 Beverage Slimmers)

Lunch

Healthy Choice Asiago Chicken Meal (2 Protein Slimmers, 1 Carb Slimmer,
 ½ Anti-Bloater/Flusher)

1 Steamfresh Singles Baby Brussels Sprouts (2 Flushers/Anti-Bloaters)

Wishbone Salad Spritzers Caesar *(optional)*, 10 sprays (½ Condiment)

1 peach (1 Flusher/Anti-Bloater)

1 cup water, 1 cup green tea (2 Beverage Slimmers)

Snack

½ cup low-fat cottage cheese (1 Protein Slimmer)

½ cup blueberries, strawberries, or blackberries (1 Flusher/Anti-Bloater)

1 cup green tea (1 Beverage Slimmer)

Dinner

Caramelized Salmon with Tropical Salsa *(See recipe page 183)*
(2½ Protein Slimmers, 1 Flusher/Anti-Bloater)

Chopped Salad with Vinaigrette Salad Dressing *(See recipe page 224)* (3 Freebies):

2 cups chopped red leaf lettuce, and spinach (2 Flushers/ Anti-Bloaters)

½ cup each chopped cucumber, tomato, zucchini (1½ Flushers/Anti-Bloaters)

1 teaspoon sunflower seeds (⅓ Mono Slimmer)

1 whole-grain roll (1 Carb Slimmer)

I Can't Believe It's Not Butter! spray for roll (1 Freebie)

2 cups water (2 Beverage Slimmers)

After-Dinner Snack *(at least an hour before bed)*

1 Skinny Cow Vanilla Fudge Bar (1 Red Light Food)

1 cup green tea (1 Beverage Slimmer)

> DAILY TOTAL: Calories 1,459, Carbohydrates 176 grams, Total Fat 31 grams, Saturated Fat 7 grams, Protein 118 grams, Fiber 36 grams, Sodium 1,277 milligrams
> 3½ Carb Slimmers, 6½ Protein Slimmers *(1 replaced 1 Red Light Food)*, ⅔ Mono Slimmers, 9½ Flushers/Anti-Bloaters, 8 Beverage Slimmers, 1 Red Light Food, 4 Freebies, ½ Condiment

Maintenance Day 10 Men

Add ¾ cup Egg Beaters to breakfast and a second roll to dinner.

> DAILY TOTAL: Calories 1,459, Carbohydrates 176 grams, Total Fat 31 grams, Saturated Fat 7 grams, Protein 118 grams, Fiber 36 grams, Sodium 1,277 milligrams
> 4½ Carb Slimmers, 8 Protein Slimmers *(1 replaced 1 Red Light Food)*, ⅔ Mono Slimmers, 9½ Flushers/Anti-Bloaters, 8 Beverage Slimmers, 1 Red Light Food, 4 Freebies, ½ Condiment

Maintenance Day 11 Women

Breakfast

The Nutrition Twins StrawBluBanana Smoothie *(See recipe page 207)*
  (2 Flushers/Anti-Bloaters, 1 Protein Slimmer)

1 cup water, 1 cup green tea (2 Beverage Slimmers)

Lunch

1 small spaghetti squash *(See recipe below)* (2 Flushers/Anti-Bloaters)

¾ cup Vegetarian Spaghetti Sauce *(See recipe page 223)* (1 Carb Slimmer) or use ½
  cup Healthy Choice Super Chunky Tomato, Mushroom & Garlic Pasta Sauce

1 tablespoon grated Parmesan (½ Condiment)

3 ounces chicken breast, baked or grilled *(dip in extra tomato sauce for flavor)*
  (1½ Protein Slimmers)

To Make: Pierce the spaghetti squash in several spots with the tip of a knife.
Heat in a microwave for 15–18 minutes on high or cook in the oven until it's
tender when you poke it with a fork. Then, let it cool for 10 minutes. Pull a
fork through the flesh to separate it into long strands and top with tomato
sauce and Parmesan cheese.

2 cups water (2 Beverage Slimmers)

Snack

1 cup Spiced Orchard Popcorn Mix *(See recipe page 203)* (1 Carb Slimmer)

3 ounces 0% Fage Greek yogurt (½ Protein Slimmer)

1 cup green tea (1 Beverage Slimmer)

Dinner

Harvest Salad with Pork *(See recipe page 212)* (2 Protein Slimmers, 2 Flushers/
  Anti-Bloaters)

1½ cups steamed mixed broccoli, squash, and carrots (1½ Flushers/Anti-Bloaters)
  sautéed with:

3 teaspoons olive oil and garlic, spritzed with juice of a lemon (1 Mono Slimmer)

½ cup wild grain rice (1 Carb Slimmer)

1 cup water, 1 cup green tea (2 Beverage Slimmers)

After-Dinner Snack *(at least an hour before bed)*

1 1.3-ounce bag Glenny's Soy Chips (2 Red Light Foods)

1 cup green tea (1 Beverage Slimmer)

> DAILY TOTAL: Calories 1,414, Carbohydrates 187 grams, Protein 86 grams, Total Fat 49 grams, Saturated Fat 9 grams, Fiber 32 grams, Sodium 1,365 milligrams
> 3 Carb Slimmers, 5 Protein Slimmers, 1 Mono Slimmer, 7½ Anti-Bloaters/Flushers *(1 replaces a Carb Slimmer)*, 8 Beverage Slimmers, 2 Red Light Foods, ½ Condiment

Maintenance Day 11 Men

Add an additional 3 ounces of grilled chicken to lunch and another ½ cup wild rice to dinner.

> DAILY TOTAL: Calories 1,630, Carbohydrates 204 grams, Protein 115 grams, Total Fat 53 grams, Saturated Fat 10 grams, Dietary Fiber 33 grams, Sodium 1,430 milligrams
> 4 Carb Slimmers, 6½ Protein Slimmers, 1 Mono Slimmer, 7½ Flushers/Anti-Bloaters *(1 replaces a Carb Slimmer)*, 8 Beverage Slimmers, 2 Red Light Foods, ½ Condiment

Maintenance Day 12 Women

Breakfast

Vans Whole Grain Original Berry Boost Waffle (1 Carb Slimmer)

1 tablespoon sugar-free syrup (2 Freebies)

½ cup blueberries, strawberries, or other berry (1 Flusher/Anti-Bloater)

6 ounces Stonyfield Farm low-fat strawberry yogurt (1½ Protein Slimmers)

1 cup water, 1 cup tea (2 Beverage Slimmers)

Lunch

Egg salad sandwich made with:

1 Toufuyan whole-wheat pita bread (1½ Carb Slimmers)

1 hard-boiled egg, mashed (1 Protein Slimmer)

1 scallion chopped (½ Flusher/Anti-Bloater)

2 teaspoons fat-free mayo (¼ Condiment)

½ cup steamed string beans (1 Flusher/Anti-Bloater)

½ cup cooked carrots (1 Flusher/Anti-Bloater)

⅓ cup vanilla ice cream (1 Red Light Food)

1 cup water, 1 cup green tea (2 Beverage Slimmers)

Snack

Peanut butter apple made with:

1 apple (1 Flusher/Anti-Bloater) dipped in:

1 tablespoon Smucker's All-Natural Peanut Butter (1 Mono Slimmer)

1 calcium-fortified diet hot chocolate (1 Condiment)

2 cups tea (2 Beverage Slimmers)

Dinner

Salad made with:

2 cups chopped Romaine lettuce (2 Flushers/Anti-Bloaters)

½ cup chopped cucumber (1 Flusher/Anti-Bloater)

½ cup chopped tomatoes (1 Flusher/Anti-Bloater)

balsamic vinegar, to taste (Unlimited)

oregano (Unlimited)

pepper (Unlimited)

lemon (Unlimited)

3 ounces sirloin steak, grilled (2 Protein Slimmers)

1 3.5-ounce (small) baked potato with lemon and pepper (1 Carb Slimmer)

1 cup steamed spinach, broccoli, and/or cauliflower, steamed with 2 cloves garlic
    (2 Flushers/Anti-Bloaters)

2 cups water (2 Beverage Slimmers)

Snack

1½ cups air-popped popcorn sprinkled with cinnamon and 20 sprays I Can't Believe It's Not Butter! spray (½ Carb Slimmer, 1 Freebie)

¾ ounce dark chocolate square (1 Red Light Food)

2 cups tea (2 Beverage Slimmers)

> DAILY TOTAL: Calories 1,409, Carbohydrates 199 grams, Total Fat 42 grams, Saturated Fat 15 grams, Protein 73 grams, Fiber 32 grams, Sodium 1,134 milligrams
> 4 Carb Slimmers, 4½ Protein Slimmers, 1 Mono Slimmer, 10½ Flushers/Anti-Bloaters, 1¼ Condiments, 10 Beverage Slimmers, 2 Red Light Foods, 3 Freebies

Maintenance Day 12 Men

Add an extra waffle to breakfast and an extra 1¾ ounces of steak to dinner.

> DAILY TOTAL: Calories 1,592, Carbohydrates 215 grams, Protein 92 grams, Total Fat 47 grams, Saturated Fat 16 grams, Fiber 33 grams, Sodium 1,329 milligrams
> 5 Carb Slimmers, 6 Protein Slimmers, 1 Mono Slimmer, 10½ Flushers/Anti-Bloaters, 1¼ Condiments, 10 Beverage Slimmers, 2 Red Light Foods, 3 Freebies

Maintenance Day 13 Women

Breakfast

½ serving Extra Spicy Potatoes *(See recipe page 215)* (¾ Carb Slimmer)

Veggie Omelet made with:

½ cup each, chopped onion, spinach, and mushrooms (1½ Flushers/Anti-Bloaters)

cooking spray (1 Freebie)

4 egg whites (1 Protein Slimmer)

½ large grapefruit (1 Flusher/Anti-Bloater)

1 cup water, 1 cup tea (2 Beverage Slimmers)

Lunch

Bean Burrito made with:

1 Thomas Sahara Wrap 100% Whole Wheat (2 Carb Slimmers)

⅓ cup Bearitos Fat Free Refried Black Beans (1 Yellow Light Food)

2 tablespoons nonfat shredded mozzarella cheese (½ Protein Slimmer)

1½ cups cooked red bell peppers, green bell peppers, and onion (3 Flushers/
Anti-Bloaters) sautéed with 1 teaspoon olive oil (⅓ Mono Slimmer)

1 cup water, 1 cup green tea (2 Beverage Slimmers)

Snack

4 Sunsweet Ones Dried Plums (1 Flusher/Anti-Bloater)

6 ounces 0% Fage Greek Yogurt (1 Protein Slimmer)

1 cup green tea (1 Beverage Slimmer)

Dinner

White Bean and Rosemary Chicken *(See recipe page 197)*
(2 Protein Slimmers, 1¼ Carb Slimmers, 1 Condiment, ½ Flusher/Anti-Bloater)

1½ cups steamed broccoli, carrots, and cauliflower (3 Flushers/Anti-Bloaters)

1 Peach and Cream Pop *(See recipe page 201)*
(½ Flusher/Anti-Bloater, ¼ Protein Slimmer)

2 cups water (2 Beverage Slimmers)

After-Dinner Snack *(at least an hour before bed)*

4 teaspoons slivered almonds (⅔ Mono Slimmer)

4 Hershey's Kisses (1 Red Light Food)

1 cup green tea (1 Beverage Slimmer)

DAILY TOTAL: Calories 1,440, Carbohydrates 206 grams, Protein 95 grams, Fat 30 grams,
Saturated Fat 8 grams, Fiber 38 grams, Sodium 1,545 milligrams
4 Carb Slimmers, 4½ Protein Slimmers, 10½ Flushers/Anti-Bloaters, 1 Mono Slimmer,
8 Beverage Slimmers, 1 Yellow Light Food, 1 Red Light Food *(extra ½ Protein instead of 1 Red
Light Food)*, 1 Condiment, 1 Freebie

Maintenance Day 13 Men

Add 4 extra egg whites and an additional half serving of potatoes to breakfast.
Add 2 tablespoons more nonfat shredded cheese to lunch.

DAILY TOTAL: Calories 1,617, Carbohydrates 224 grams, Total Fat 31 grams, Saturated Fat 8 grams, Protein 122 grams, Fiber 40 grams, Sodium 1,849 milligrams
4¾ Carb Slimmers, 6 Protein Slimmers, 10½ Flushers/Anti-Bloaters, 1 Mono Slimmer, 8 Beverage Slimmers, 1 Yellow Light Food, 1 Red Light Food *(extra ½ protein instead of other Red Light Food)*, 1 Condiment, 1 Freebie

Maintenance Day 14 Women

Breakfast

Zucchini and Tomato Frittata *(See recipe page 208)* (1¼ Protein Slimmers,
    ½ Flusher/Anti-Bloater)

1 Pepperidge Farm Whole Grain 100% Whole Wheat English Muffin
    (1½ Carb Slimmers)

10 sprays I Can't Believe It's Not Butter! spray or 1 tablespoon sugar-free jelly
    (1 Freebie)

1 cup water, 1 cup green tea (2 Beverage Slimmers)

Lunch

1 Gardenburger Black Bean Chipotle Veggie Burger (1 Protein Slimmer)

½ ounce nonfat cheddar cheese (½ Protein Slimmer)

Several lettuce leaves to make a bed for the veggie burger (¼ Flusher/Anti-Bloater)

¾ cup fresh corn (1 Carb Slimmer)

1 cup coleslaw made with:

1 cup shredded cabbage (1 Flusher/Anti-Bloater)

1 teaspoon caraway seeds (Unlimited)

1 tablespoon fat-free mayonnaise (½ Condiment)

1 cup baby carrots (1 Flusher/Anti-Bloater)

2 cups seltzer (2 Beverage Slimmers)

Mid-Afternoon Snack

Orange (1 Flusher/Anti-Bloater)

6-ounce yogurt *(plain nonfat or any fat-free, light yogurt)* (1 Protein Slimmer)

15 pistachios (½ Mono Slimmer)

1 cup green tea (1 Beverage Slimmer)

Dinner

Chopped Salad made with:

½ cup each chopped tomato, romaine lettuce, cucumber, zucchini, carrots
(2½ Flushers/Anti-Bloaters)

1½ teaspoons olive oil and vinegar, to taste (½ Mono Slimmer)

Creamy Chicken Penne *(See recipe page 184)*
(1½ Carb Slimmers, 1½ Protein Slimmers, ½ Flusher/Anti-Bloater)

2 cups water (2 Beverage Slimmers)

After-Dinner Snack (at least one hour before bed)

1 peach chopped (1 Flusher/Anti-Bloater) and mixed in:

1 cup fat-free frozen yogurt (2 Red Light Foods)

1 cup green tea (1 Beverage Slimmer)

> DAILY TOTAL: Calories 1,431, Carbohydrates 214 grams, Total Fat 34 grams, Saturated Fat
> 6 grams, Protein 78 grams, Fiber 27 grams, Sodium 1,621 milligrams
> 4 Carb Slimmers, 5¼ Protein Slimmers, 1 Mono Slimmer, 7¾ Flushers/Anti-Bloaters,
> 8 Beverage Slimmers, 2 Red Light Foods, ½ Condiment, 1 Freebie

Maintenance Day 14 Men

Add an extra ¾ cup of fresh corn at lunch. Add an extra 3 ounces of chicken to
the Creamy Chicken Penne.

> DAILY TOTAL: Calories 1,644, Carbohydrates 236 grams, Protein 102 grams, Total Fat 37
> grams, Saturated Fat 7 grams, Fiber 31 grams, Sodium 1,689 milligrams
> 5 Carb Slimmers, 6¾ Protein Slimmers, 1 Mono Slimmer, 7¾ Flushers/Anti-Bloaters,
> 8 Beverage Slimmers, 2 Red Light Foods, ½ Condiment, 1 Freebie

Chapter 8

Red Light Foods: Pluggers, Bloaters, Chubbers, and Flabbers

In this chapter we give you the low-down on the Red Light foods—the worst weight-loss saboteurs and the biggest diet derailers. While you avoided the Red Light foods on the Jumpstart Plan, the Maintenance Plan allows 2 small servings of Red Light foods per day.

A Red Light food serving is generally equal to 100 calories (condiments and convenience foods are exceptions to the 100-calorie servings; you'll see their serving sizes in Appendix III). You can have up to two of most of the items on the Red Light foods list each day. However, some foods are extreme Bloaters, with 600 milligrams of sodium or more per serving, so they will count as both of your Red Light foods for the day.

Although we've grouped the Red Light foods into four categories—Pluggers, Bloaters, Chubbers, and Flabbers—many will fall into more than one category. By understanding which foods bloat you, make you flabby, or cause you to be constipated, you will better understand your body and learn how to make it look and feel its best. For instance, if you know that you tend to be constipated, avoid choosing Pluggers as your Red Light foods. On the other hand, for example, if you tend to have swollen hands or ankles, or a distended stomach after having a salty food like soy sauce, avoid choosing Bloaters as your Red Light foods. In this way, you can use the chart below to your advantage.

Red Light Foods	Where You Find Them	Why They're Bad for Your Body
Pluggers	Foods low in fiber and fluid and high in fat and/or refined flour like white bread, fatty cuts of red meat, and full-fat cheese	Constipating foods that plug you up and result in a nearly instant weight gain
Bloaters	Salt-laden foods and condiments like pickles, pretzels, and deli meats, and beverages such as alcohol. Sugary foods like jelly beans also cause water retention and bloating	Water-retaining foods that create a bloated, distended belly; they lead to salt toxicity and a bigger, prematurely aged, and damaged body
Chubbers	Foods loaded with artery-clogging and aging saturated fats or trans fat, such as ice cream, whole milk, and butter	Typically not high in salt, yet they're belt-bursting foods because they contain high amounts of fat that chub your body and prematurely age you.
Flabbers	The worst of the worst—they're a double whammy: foods loaded with both salt and artery-clogging fat, such as French fries, baked goods, and most fast foods	Contribute to a flabby body and negatively impact nearly every aspect of health

As we mentioned, in the Maintenance phase you're allowed to have 2 Red Light foods daily—the trick is to keep the portion sizes small so that any damage they do is minimal and easily balanced by the Green Light foods in this plan.

For real Red Light doozies—like some fast foods that have more fat and sodium than you should get in a day—you'll limit the food to 300 calories' worth, which means you won't eat the whole thing. You'll also only allow such a damaging food once a week. You'll count that food as both of your Red Light foods and 1 Yellow Light food. Some frozen entrées also have too many calories (some have much more than 300 calories) and likewise, you won't be able to eat the whole frozen entrée. Also, for some fast foods, you'll have to eat less than half.

Table 5 lists Red Light foods and their qualifications. Most portions are listed as 100 calories and count as 1 Red Light food.

Table 5: Red Light Food Qualifications

Foods	If Your Food Has Any *One* of These Qualifications It Is a Red Light Food	Red Light Servings
Bread (Stick to ≤120 calories per serving (made from whole or refined grains)	≥400 mg sodium per serving *or* ≤2 grams fiber	1 Red Light Food 1 Red Light Food
Cereals: Stick to ≤120 calories per serving (made from whole or refined grains)	≥400 mg sodium per serving *or* cold cereals ≤5 grams fiber *or* hot cereals ≤ 3 grams fiber *or* ≥8 grams sugars	1 Red Light Food 1 Red Light Food 1 Red Light Food 1 Red Light Food
Fresh or canned starchy vegetables, tomato sauce, legumes (beans) (50–100 calories) (Rinse all beans and vegetables)	600–800 mg sodium per serving	2 Red Light Foods

Table 5: Red Light Food Qualifications *(continued)*

Foods	If Your Food Has Any *One* of These Qualifications It Is a Red Light Food	Red Light Servings
Cheeses, Milk (and Soy Milk), and Other Dairy Products: regular and reduced fat, *not* low fat or fat free (limit to 100 calories, generally 1 ounce for cheese)	≥3 grams of fat in a serving *or* ≥ more than 1 gram saturated fat *or* Yogurt ≥30 grams of added sugar	1 Red Light Food 1 Red Light Food 1 Red Light Food
Meat, Poultry	≥140 mg sodium in single, raw ingredient per 2-ounce serving	1 Red Light Food
Canned Fish and Poultry (per 2-ounce serving, choose in water only)	600–800 mg per 2-ounce serving	2 Red Light Foods
Deli Meats	Per 2-ounce serving: 600–800 mg sodium *or* ≥3 grams fat	2 Red Light Foods 1 Red Light Food
Fats, Oils, Spreads: butter, margarine, shortening, palm oils (Limit to 100 calories)	>140 mg sodium per serving *or* >1 gram saturated and trans fat combined	1 Red Light Food 1 Red Light Food
Salted Seeds, Nuts, Nut Butters, Olives (Limit to 100-calorie portions, 100 calories = approximately 11 nuts; approximately 18 small or 9 large olives)	Salted nuts and olives ≥600 mg sodium per serving	2 Red Light Foods
Fresh and canned vegetables, fruits, and non-starchy tomato sauce (less than 50 calories)	600–800 mg sodium per serving *or* Fruits canned in syrup	2 Red Light Foods
Condiments (See Appendix II, List E)		

Table 5: Red Light Food Qualifications *(continued)*

Foods	If Your Food Has Any *One* of These Qualifications It Is a Red Light Food	Red Light Servings
MISCELLANEOUS		
Alcohol	(See 100 Calorie Serving Size on Page 276)	1 Red Light Food
Sugary Candy (Limit to 100 calories): Gummy Bears, Twizzlers, etc.	See Page 275	1 Red Light Food
Beverages (100 calories serving)	≥60 mg sodium per serving	2 Red Light Foods
Convenience Foods: entrees, sandwiches, pre-pared meats, soups, main dishes, meals including frozen entrees and snacks like pretzels		
	600–800 mg sodium ≤200 calories, especially bad if ≥ 2 grams saturated fat *or* <3 grams fiber	2 Red Light Foods
	800–1000 mg sodium ≤200 calories, especially bad if ≥ 2 grams saturated fat *or* <3 grams fiber	2 Red Light Foods and 1 Yellow Light Food
	600–800 mg sodium 220–300 calories (300 calories maximum)	2 Red Light Foods and 1 Yellow Light Food
	800–1,000 mg sodium 220–300 calories (300 calories maximum)	2 Red Light Foods and 1 Yellow Light Food, limit to once a week

Now that you know the basics of the Pluggers, Bloaters, Flabbers, and Chubbers, we'll give you more details so you can fine-tune your diet and get your body in tip-top shape.

The Nitty-Gritty of the Pluggers

Pluggers are processed foods such as Cream of Wheat and white bread, neither of which are made from whole grains, and both of which are stripped of nutrients and fiber. Full-fat cheeses and other full-fat dairy products are also considered Pluggers because they lead to constipation and contribute to weight gain. Aside from making you look and feel bloated, constipation makes you downright uncomfortable. Plus, when you're constipated, food lingers in your colon without getting flushed out, which is why Pluggers can cause nearly instant weight gain.

For the most part, Pluggers also fall under one of the other Red Light food categories, so they were off-limits on the Jumpstart Plan. On the Maintenance Plan, some Pluggers are allowed. When you eat a Plugger, you should combat the damage with fibrous foods such as strawberries, spinach, or oatmeal (Flushers or Carbohydrate Slimmers) that prevent constipation. The most common cause of constipation? A diet that is low in fiber and fluid and high in fat.

The Most Common Pluggers

- White bread
- Refined foods: all refined, white flour foods, like cereals, tortillas, and pastas not made with the whole grain
- Sugar and sugary foods
- Cheese (Full-fat cheese is a Red Light food and should be avoided, but low-fat and nonfat cheeses (despite being constipating and somewhat plugging) are Slimmers

- Rich, high-calorie, low-fiber foods such as ice cream and butter
- High-fat meats like bacon, salami, lamb, rib steak, etc.
- Low-fiber processed snacks such as chips and pizza
- Low-fiber frozen dinners
- Instant mashed potatoes
- Iron supplements (Speak to your doctor or registered dietitian if you take them and tend to suffer from constipation)
- Calcium supplements without added magnesium
- Not enough water or other fluids
- Sedentary lifestyle
- Laxatives (Surprisingly, although they help fight constipation, they frequently do more harm than good. They're easy to get hooked on, and they kill friendly, necessary bacteria in your gut, reducing absorption of nutrients and important vitamins and minerals.)

The Nitty-Gritty of the Bloaters

Salt-loaded Bloaters include vegetable and chicken broths, miso soup, or a teriyaki stir-fry. They immediately create a bloated, distended belly and lead to salt toxicity and a bigger, prematurely aged and damaged body. Even if you are lean, these foods can make your clothes feel tight and can make you feel like you have a layer of flab under your skin. In general, Bloaters are low in fat but high in sodium, containing 100 milligrams or more per serving. You'll find that many Bloaters count as both of your Red Light foods for the day because they have more than 600 milligrams of sodium.

You'll always have at least one Anti-Bloater any time you eat a Bloater. Use Appendix III as your guide to find 100-calorie Bloater portions and their respective sodium ranges. Make it a habit to always check the Nutrition Facts panel (see chapter 4) of any Bloater to try to avoid Bloaters that qualify as 2 Red Light foods. Ensure that your Bloater doesn't contain more sodium than the range provided in Appendix III. If your food (deli meats, canned soups, etc.) has even more sodium than we list, switch brands.

Below we tell you why some unexpected foods are Bloaters—this way you'll know to have your eye out for them and how to choose the least damaging ones. If you frequently eat any of these foods, as you follow our plan and scale back on them, you'll see your body undergo an incredible transformation.

CANADIAN BACON

Canadian bacon is actually a lean meat, but it is loaded with sodium. However, it's much better than regular bacon. Be sure to stick to the 2-ounce serving size and check the Nutrition Facts on the label. Different brands can vary by more than 100 milligrams of sodium per serving.

CANNED BEANS

Although beans are excellent for you, if you don't rinse canned varieties to wash away the extra salt, you'll surely swallow a Bloater as you'll add an extra 600 milligrams or more of sodium to your day—and that's only for a ½-cup serving. Be sure to avoid beans with added pork or bacon and beans that are refried, except fat-free and low-fat refried beans. Remember to read the labels. You might be surprised to see that Taco Bell Fat Free Refried Beans has at least ten milligrams less sodium per ½-cup serving than the Old El Paso brand (460 milligrams versus 570 milligrams).

CANNED TUNA AND OTHER FISH, SHELLFISH

All fish start as Protein Slimmers, but once they're dried, fried, canned in oil, or flavored, the sodium (or fat) will cost you. Watch the fish steaks such as Chicken of the Sea Fish Steaks in Hot Sauce—it's a super Bloater with 860 milligrams of sodium in just about 3 ounces; you'll have to count it as both of your Yellow Light and your Red Light food servings for the day. Note: Always choose fish canned in water; fish canned in oil is very high in calories because it absorbs the extra oil.

CEREALS

Generally, refined and processed cereals such as Rice Krispies, corn flakes, or puffed cereals are Bloaters. They may be low in sugar, but they are high in salt. And because they are refined, they lack fiber and are digested quickly. You may be hungry within one to two hours of eating them. But that will be the least of your problems—you'll also likely feel quite bloated from the excess salt they contain (more than 400 milligrams of sodium in a serving). More than likely, you'll be constipated from such fiber-lacking cereals as well. A cereal that is a Bloater will also be a Flabber if it has more than 140 calories and 3 grams of fat in a serving. Instead, choose cereals like oatmeal, Kashi Go Lean, or Post Shredded Wheat.

CHICKEN

If your raw chicken is injected with sodium (it will say "sodium" on the label), it's a Bloater. Find a better option like Perdue Fit & Easy Fresh Ground Chicken Breast or Harvestland's skinless chicken breasts.

REFINED AND WHITE BREADS, PITAS, WRAPS

Surprisingly, these processed grains are often as high, if not higher, in sodium than many chips and snack foods. For instance, there are much better options, like Pepperidge Farm Stoneground 100% Whole Wheat or Sara Lee's 45 Calories and Delightful—100% Multi-Grain or 100% Whole Wheat with Honey (see our list on page 243 for brands of breads that are Carbohydrate Slimmers).

Salad Dressing Tricks

When adding dressing to your salad, keep a measuring spoon handy to use until you are able to eyeball both 1- and 2-tablespoon portions. Better yet, try one of these tricks:

- Keep your dressing on the side and dip your fork in it before you stab each bite of salad. You'll get great flavor but fewer calories and sodium.
- Thin out thick salad dressing with a little water or skim milk to dilute the calories and salt.
- Put your dressing in a spray bottle and spritz it on your salad. You'll still get the flavor with minimal fat and calories

Some of the best dressings are those you make yourself. Try mixing a few tablespoons of balsamic vinegar with a teaspoon of high-quality fruity olive oil. You can add lemon or garlic, too.

SALAD DRESSING

If a dressing contains more than 240 milligrams of sodium per serving, it's a Bloater. (And if it is a creamy dressing, such as bleu cheese or ranch, that is high in artery-clogging saturated fat, it's likely a Flabber, too.) Limit your Red Light dressing servings to 100 calories. And remember, you can make any dressing count as a Condiment on the Maintenance Plan if you stick to an amount that is less than 60 calories and 240 milligrams of sodium.

SUGARY FOODS

Although sugary foods don't necessarily contain sodium, they do cause bloating. Like salt, sugar attracts water to dilute it. Sugary foods contain very few, if any, nutrients. Instead they're usually plugging, high-calorie, and often high-fat foods, too.

The Skinniest Treats

Although sweets and snack foods are not health food, everyone should be allowed to indulge now and then. Ultimately, treats help so that you don't feel deprived and so that you stay on track. You can still indulge on the Maintenance Plan: Just choose wisely. Count the item as one of your 100-calorie servings of Red Light foods. Here's a list of our favorite Skinniest Treats. Those that aren't individually packaged are listed with their 100-calorie serving size.

- Skinny Cow Ice Cream Sandwiches, Cones & Ice Cream Bars
- 4 Hershey's kisses
- ½ cup nonfat frozen yogurt/ice cream
- 2 Hershey's miniatures
- 1 to 2 small Peppermint Patties
- 1 cup nonfat pudding
- 1 small slice of angel food cake *(1 ounce)*
- Soy chips *(individual serving bag)*
- Baked Lays *(1 ounce, 11 chips)*
- Glenny's Low-Fat Apple Cinnamon Soy Chips *(½ 1.3-ounce bag)*
- Utz Organic Seven Whole Grain Pretzel Sticks *(1 ounce)*
- Snikiddy Chocolate Chip Bites *(4 cookies)*
- Snikiddy Oatmeal Chocolate Bites *(4 cookies)*

 Did you know? One and a half ounces of chocolate Hershey's Kisses *(9 kisses)* has 230 calories and 13 grams of fat, while the same amount of fresh dates *(5 dates)* rolled in cocoa powder has just 125 calories and less than 1 gram of fat.

CONDIMENTS

If your favorite condiment is on the Red Light foods list, don't panic. There's good news. You don't have to count your condiment as a Bloater if you consume it in a smaller amount. For example, although 2 tablespoons of ketchup has 380 milligrams of sodium and counts as a Bloater, you can have 2 teaspoons of ketchup (just 125 milligrams of sodium) and count it as a Condiment instead. This means that you'll have a Bloater serving to spare. More good news: some condiments have low-calorie and low-sodium counterparts. There's low-sodium mustard such as Nathan's Original Coney Island Deli Style Mustard and Westbrae No Salt Added Stoneground Mustard, low-sodium ketchup such as Heinz No Salt Added Ketchup, and even low-sodium hot wing sauce such as Mr. Spice Hot Wing! Sauce.

Check out some other lower-sodium condiments and their serving sizes in the Maintenance Plan foods on page 266–270.

Top Condiment Choices

- **Balsamic vinegar.** Two teaspoons has 14 calories, 0 grams fat, and 2 milligrams sodium. (You don't even have to count it as a Freebie!)

- **Mustard.** One teaspoon has 10 calories, 0 grams fat, and 100 milligrams sodium.

- **Pickle relish.** One tablespoon has 21 calories, 0 grams fat, and 109 milligrams sodium.

- **Horseradish.** Two teaspoons has 4 calories, 0 grams fat, and 10 milligrams sodium.

- **Low-sodium light mayonnaise.** One-half tablespoon has approximately 17 calories, 1.3 grams fat, and 27 milligrams sodium.

(cont'd on page 155)

> • **Lemon.** Juice from ½ lemon has 8 calories, 0 grams fat, and 1 milligram sodium. (You don't even have to count it as a Freebie!)

Don't see your favorite condiment on the list? Check its Nutrition Facts label to see if it has less than 240 milligrams of sodium per serving. Remember, just as with salad dressings, you can make any condiment a Green Light food [or acceptable on the Maintenance Plan] if you adjust the portion to meet the calorie (less than 60) and sodium (less than 240 milligrams) guidelines.

ALCOHOL

Although alcohol is not salt-laden, it is a bona fide Bloater. Beer especially creates flatulence and stomach distention. All alcohol causes puffiness under your eyes. Use your food journal to record how your stomach (and your face) responds to alcohol. Not only is alcohol high in calories, which clearly contributes to weight gain (alcohol has 7 calories per gram, making it nearly as calorie dense as fat, which has 9 calories per gram), it also doesn't satisfy appetite, so it's easy to drink a lot of calories without realizing it. Making matters worse, alcohol makes you hungrier and lowers your inhibitions, so you eat more while you are already getting excess calories from drinking. Yes, alcohol causes fat gain everywhere, and most notably in the abdominal area for the majority of people.

What's more, the body has no storage capacity for alcohol like it does for carbohydrates and fats. And because the body isn't designed to metabolize it, alcohol disrupts the functioning of your liver. It is the liver's job to package fatty acids (triglycerides) so that they can be sent out of the body to prevent creating bodily harm, including a fatty liver. When alcohol is present, the liver has to stop its usual job and break down the alcohol to rid your body of this harmful toxin. This means that fatty acids will accumulate (fat accumulation on the liver can be seen after a single night of heavy drinking). As you can imagine, a liver clogged with fat cannot function properly, which results in liver damage. And while the liver is metabolizing the alcohol, the utilization of fats, carbohydrates, and protein has to be temporarily suppressed. Yes, alcohol puts fat metabolism on hold.

 If you choose alcohol as your Red Light Bloater serving for the day, stick to a drink with the least calories—light beer, reduced- or no-sugar coolers, or reduced-alcohol wine. Cocktails are double whammies because you get calories from both the alcohol and the sugary syrup or juice that's added to the mix.

The Skinny on Fat

Think all that matters for being healthy and losing weight is the salt in your food? Think again! Our diet plan may be based on lowering sodium, but you can't forget the importance of limiting fat—especially the saturated and trans kinds—in your diet. You may know something about fat, but let's refresh your memory. Dietary fat is one of the three most important nutrients you need to have a healthy diet (the other two are carbohydrates and protein). However, the type of fat and how much of it you have are both key factors. Total fat intake should be no more than 30 percent of your calories—that means that if you are on a 1,200-calorie plan, you should have no more than 40 grams of fat per day. Of the 30 percent total fat you should have per day, most should come from mono- and polyunsaturated fats, which have positive health effects, and less than 10 percent should come from saturated fat, which can be damaging to your health.

In the past, saturated fat was considered the worst culprit in foods, and food manufacturers reduced their use of saturated fats but were able to keep the great taste of their foods by adding trans fats. After many years of research we now know that trans fats are even worse for you than saturated fats. Similar to saturated fats, trans fats increase the LDL "bad" cholesterol, but on top of that trans fats lower the HDL "good" cholesterol; so you get two times the negative impact on your heart health by eating foods that contain them. What exactly are trans fats? They are manmade fats created by adding hydrogen to unsaturated fats, such as vegetable oils, which makes them saturated. Food manufacturers started this hydrogenation process to extend the shelf life of certain foods, including crackers, cakes, shortening, fried foods (like doughnuts), and even some types of peanut butter (not the natural ones, which are *great* for you!).

Good News for Potato Chip Lovers: Did you know that often a serving of potato chips contains less sodium per serving than a slice of bread? That's because they sprinkle the salt on the surface so it hits your tongue first. Our favorite chips are the Lays, which are made with three simple ingredients—potatoes, salt, and healthier oils (so there's no trans fat or cholesterol). So although chips certainly aren't a health food and should be limited, take this as a lesson to learn about the power of sodium on the surface of a food.

Weight-Saving SWAP
- Replace your nightly cup of ice cream with a Skinny Cow ice cream sandwich and save nearly 26 pounds a year.
- Choose turkey subs instead of tuna twice a week and save over 7 pounds a year.
- Swap the half and half in your coffee for skim milk or 1% milk, and save 6 pounds a year.

The Nitty-Gritty of the Chubbers

Chubbers are foods like butter, whole milk, some full-fat cheeses, cream, ice cream, and coconut that are loaded with saturated fat or trans fat that clogs your arteries, ages you prematurely, and causes weight gain. While they don't contain high amounts of salt (generally

You may be surprised to see coconut counted as a Chubber, but ounce for ounce, coconut oil delivers more artery-clogging saturated fat than butter, lard, or margarine. A 2-ounce piece of fresh coconut has more than 13 grams of saturated fat—nearly two-thirds the recommended daily limit!

less than 240 milligrams per serving), they will add to the numbers on your scale.

Many Chubbers are also Pluggers, promoting not only body fat gain, but constipation, too. What's more, in our society of overly processed foods, there aren't too many foods that exist as just Chubbers—most prepared foods that are Chubbers have been plumped up with salt, making them the ultimate of the Red Light foods—Flabbers. The good news is that there are some easy ways to avoid eating Chubbers, since most of them have healthier alternatives. Consider these swaps:

Weight-Saving SWAP

• Choose low-fat or fat-free cheeses instead of the regular versions.
• Use I Can't Believe It's Not Butter! Light, Brummel & Brown, or Promise Spread Light instead of butter.
• Use skim or 1% milk instead of whole milk.
• Enjoy low-fat ice cream instead of the full-fat variety.

By making these swaps, you'll save yourself a Red Light food. Better yet, you'll be saving your waistline and your heart.

The Nitty-Gritty of the Flabbers

Flabbers are the worst of the worst when it comes to weight loss and health. Flabbers are Red Light foods such as fried foods and pastries that contribute to a flabby body and negatively impact nearly every aspect of your health. Flabbers are both high in artery-clogging fat and in bloating salt and ideally should be avoided during both the Jumpstart Plan and the Maintenance Plan (and for the rest of your life, for that matter). However, since this plan is realistic, we do allow for some Flabbers in the Maintenance Plan.

The Most Common Flabbers

- Baked goods, such as pastries, cakes, cookies, pies, doughnuts, sweet rolls
- Buttermilk
- Creamy soups and chowders (canned or dehydrated)
- Cured fatty meats, such as bacon, sausage, ham, bologna, salami, and smoked beef
- Fast-food meals
- Fish (frozen prebreaded and fried, or canned in oil)
- Frankfurters, wieners, hot dogs
- Fried foods
- Frozen entrées with more than 10 grams of fat and more than 600 milligrams of sodium
- Full-fat dairy products
- Meat pie, goulash, beef chili
- Pizza
- Potato chips, buttered popcorn, and crackers such as Ritz
- Refined, cheesy pastas like lasagna, manicotti, ravioli, macaroni and cheese
- Salad dressings, especially creamy ones
- Tacos, enchiladas, tamales, burritos, tostados
- Quiche and soufflés

Hopefully avoiding or scaling back on Red Light foods will come naturally for you as you fill up on the Green Light foods and see amazing results. Your new way of eating will soon become second nature: feeling lean, refreshed, and energized will be so much a part of who you are that you will continue on your path to a trim, fit, and healthy body!

Chapter 9

Move It and Lose It

Of course you're going to see fabulous results from the dietary changes you are making. Reducing your sodium and calorie intake will help you lose weight and lower your risk of high blood pressure, heart disease, and countless other diseases, but you won't burn nearly as many calories or see the results as quickly as you will if you exercise. We know—many people don't want to exercise because they think of it as a chore or hard work. But without it, you're missing half of the weight-loss equation. Add exercise to the plan, and you'll quickly lose pounds, fat, and the bloat! You'll love having a body that feels tight and toned—something only exercise, not diet alone, can do for you. Only exercise can give a lift to both your spirits and your tush. And as you're exercising, you'll sweat out salt and toxins, leaving you feeling slim and full of energy. No diet plan would be complete without exercise, so get ready, because you're about to embark on the physical component to your weight-loss success!

You may think that the sole benefit of exercise is to help you lose weight and get in shape. Although it does both of those things, exercise can help with so much more. Not only will you feel more energized and less stiff, but you'll also sleep better, get sick less often, and have better posture. You'll also start to feel better about yourself, and as studies have shown, have an uplifted mood. And, as if those benefits weren't enough, exercise will also improve your coordination, balance, and heart—your most important muscle. Finally, let's not forget about what exercise does for your blood pressure: 60 to 90 minutes a week of exercise can significantly lower your blood pressure, which leads to less risk of hypertension. Once you get over the initial hurdle of starting to exercise, it gets easier. You will begin to get into better shape quickly and the exercise actually will start to feel good—so good in fact, that before you know it you may even start to crave the movement. You'll also love the mood boost and endorphin rush you get, and you'll feel happier and more positive knowing you're doing something really good for yourself. Plus, for most people, exercise will mean just moving your body. Keep it simple and fun—remember that even just walking is considered exercise—and it certainly burns a lot more calories and gets your heart beating faster than sitting at a desk.

Now that you know how integral exercise is to your weight-loss success, are you all pumped up and ready to begin? But wait just a minute—before you go out there for a speed walk or head to that spin class, make sure you check with your doctor. Whether you've been a gym rat for years or it's your first time getting on the bike, it's always a good idea to get the green light from your doctor before you begin any new exercise regimen. No matter how old you are, what condition your body is in, or what level of ability you're at, it's important to ask your doctor what you can and can't do. Once your physician gives you the go-ahead, sprint for the finish line!

Your Cardio Plan

Now for the fun part! Cardiovascular activity (also known as aerobic exercise or "cardio," for short) is the exercise that burns the most calories while you do it and is going to help you to slim your body and sweat out the bloat. You want to aim for at least 30 minutes every day, especially during the ten-day Jumpstart Plan—no excuses! If you're new to exercise, you may want to start out at whatever pace allows you to get the minimum 30 minutes of exercise daily. As your fitness improves you can move faster for the 30 minutes and aim to work your way up to 45 minutes or even an hour several days a week for maximum results. If 60 minutes is unrealistic for you, then be sure to get the minimum 30 minutes daily, always having a goal in mind to aim for more. After the initial ten-day period, when you enter the Maintenance Plan, you can drop your cardio to six days a week. Keep in mind that your exercise doesn't need to exhaust you—in fact, it should be something you like to do and find enjoyable.

If you don't belong to a gym or haven't exercised in a long time, start by walking for 30 minutes a day—even if it just means that you'll be stepping out of your front door and walking briskly for 15 minutes before turning back. That's fine with us. Just be sure to get that activity in each day. For an added bonus, take the stairs at work, do jumping jacks during the commercial breaks of your favorite TV show, and—yes, you've heard this one before—take the furthest spot in the parking lot. Although these aren't exactly long-lasting calorie-blasting activities, they are bonus steps. Moving burns more calories than sitting still, and this will all accumulate and contribute to your body-fat loss. Even housework can count as an activity—after all, you are expending energy when you clean your toilets! However, don't let this be the substitute for cardiovascular exercise—count it as a bonus, too. The goal is to get as many "bonuses" as possible in your day—this is especially critical if you aren't able to meet the exercise recommendations. As you progress, you can practice some more intense forms of cardio, such as jogging around a track, riding your bike, or doing a home exercise video. The following chart shows the approximate calories burned during 30 minutes of some activities. The calories burned are based on weight, and notice that at a higher weight you burn more because it takes more energy to move a heavier mass.

Activity	Your Approximate Weight (in Pounds)					
	110	130	150	170	190	215
Aerobic dancing: Easy	144	177	201	225	252	291
Intense	201	237	276	312	348	396
Car Washing	105	123	144	165	177	207
Cycling:						
Leisurely (9.4 mph)	150	177	204	231	258	294
Racing, fast	255	300	345	390	435	498
Free-weight lifting	129	150	174	198	222	252
Gardening: Digging	139	222	258	291	324	369
Raking	129	150	174	195	219	249
Housework: Dusting	99	114	132	148	164	189
Laundry	102	117	135	156	173	192
Vacuuming	132	156	180	201	225	255
Running (on flat surface):						
11 min 30 sec/mile	204	240	276	315	351	399
9 min/mile	291	342	393	447	498	567
7 min/mile	366	417	468	522	573	642
Walking (leisurely, outdoors)	120	141	161	186	207	234
Yoga	93	111	126	144	159	183

Other Cardio Activities You Can Do

- **Get jumping.** Jumping rope isn't just for kids. Get out that rope and show your kids how it's done.

- **Shake your groove.** Dancing doesn't have to be saved for a wedding. Take a dance class or turn on your iPod and shake a leg.

- **"Ten-hut."** March in place as you watch your favorite TV show or when you need a break to stretch your legs at the office. Every little movement counts!

- **Give Fido some exercise.** Take your dog out for a walk and speed it up—dogs need exercise, too.

If you've been working out regularly for some time, you may need to step up your workouts a notch to make sure your cardio plan is intense enough.

To ensure you're getting the most out of your workouts, make sure that your heart rate is in your "target heart rate zone." This way you won't be exercising too intensely or too lightly. Your target heart rate is the number of times that your heart should beat each minute while you're exercising. It should be 60–75% of your maximum heart rate. See the chart on the following page to find your target heart rate.

In order to determine your heart rate, first take your pulse. Finding your radial pulse: using your middle and index fingers, locate your pulse on the thumb-side of your wrist. Press lightly and count your pulse for 15 seconds starting with zero. Keep exercising while you're taking your pulse, just move at a slower pace. Use the chart on the following page to determine your 15-second count.

Target Heart Rate							
		Target Zone			15-Second Count		
Age	**Max HR**	**60%**	**70%**	**80%**	**60%**	**70%**	**80%**
20	200	120	140	160	30	35	40
25	195	117	137	156	29	34	39
30	190	114	133	152	29	33	38
35	185	111	130	148	28	32	37
40	180	108	126	144	27	32	36
45	175	105	123	140	26	31	35
50	170	102	119	136	26	30	34
55	165	99	116	132	25	29	33
60	160	96	112	128	24	28	32
65+	155	93	109	124	23	27	31

Or maybe you're just not seeing results from what you're doing. Often when you do the same exercises every day you get accustomed to your routine, and it's no longer a challenge. When that happens, it means it's time to shake things up a bit, and one great way to do that is through interval training. Interval training consists of short, high-intensity periods of exercise alternated with low-intensity recovery periods. The higher-intensity exercise challenges your body in new ways, which means you'll burn more calories and fat. The low-intensity recovery periods, also known as *rest intervals,* are important because they ensure that your high-intensity intervals are done at an optimal intensity. Without the rest intervals you'll only be able to work at a medium intensity for the full duration of your exercise—which is no different than what you were doing before. For example, if your routine is to run at 5 mph for 30 minutes, interval training would change this routine to running at 6.5 mph for 3 minutes, reducing the speed to 4 mph for 3 minutes, increasing the speed back to 6 or 7 mph for 3 minutes, reducing the speed back to 5 or 6 mph for 3 minutes, and so on for a total of 30 minutes. As you progress, you can change your intervals around to be more challenging, which will only lead to better results and reduce boredom!

Work Those Muscles

Now that you've got the cardio regimen down, let's move on to the strength-training component. Strength training is super important because it helps to keep your muscles taut as you lose that fat! Strengthening your muscles not only tightens and firms them, it also boosts your metabolism. Muscles are calorie-blasters—the more muscle you have, the more calories your body burns, even while you sleep. However, if you aren't already performing strength-training exercises, don't start until phase 2 of the plan, after you've completed the Jumpstart phase. Those first ten days are solely to help you lose weight and burn fat and calories, and that's just what cardio does for you, so you want to put all your energy into it. If strength training is already a part of your regular exercise routine, then continue as you have been even during the Jumpstart phase. After the Jumpstart phase, when you have focused on doing your cardio every day, you can start adding in strength training—even if you're a beginner. Aim to do strength training three times a week and include all your major muscle groups. If you've never weight trained before and you are a woman who is worried you'll get "bulky," don't fret—weight training improves your muscle strength and tone without making you look like a body builder. Women don't have enough of the hormone testosterone, which builds those big, bulky muscles. Strength training also improves your posture (so you'll look longer and leaner), helps you with your balance, decreases your risk of osteoporosis, and will help you perform everyday activities, such as carrying your groceries and lifting things.

There are so many benefits of strength training that just imagining your great results should be enough to inspire you to do it now! Three times a week you want to work your back, chest, legs, abdomen and arms—all of your major muscle groups. It's important though that you don't work the same muscles on consecutive days—take a day off between workouts to allow your muscles time to repair and rebuild themselves. If you're new to weight training, don't push it the first time you lift weights. Just because some big macho guy at the gym is lifting 50-pound weights doesn't mean that's the right weight for you. Start with what you think you can lift, whether it's 5, 8, or 10 pounds, and as you get stronger you'll lift more. For every exercise, do 3 sets of 10 repetitions. In other words, each set of an exercise should consist of lifting the weight 10 times. If you don't feel challenged by the tenth repetition, the weight is too light, and you need to use a heavier one. Ideally, by your last repetition in each set, you will feel as if you couldn't do another one. After completing each set, rest for 1 minute before starting the next set.

If you're already doing strength training, and you've been following the same regimen for a long time, you may want to try some new exercises or do some circuit training to mix it up. Challenging your muscles in a new way will give your body a boost, and you'll build more lean, calorie-blasting muscle and burn more calories. When you circuit train you quickly move from one muscle group to another without resting in between. You'll end up working more muscles in less time and being more efficient. The key is to work opposing muscles back to back. For example, after you work your hamstrings, immediately do a set of quadriceps exercises; or after you finish working your biceps, work your triceps. If you belong to a gym, ask a qualified personal trainer for assistance in circuit training the first time you do it—they'll guide you on which machines to use and how to use them effectively. If you don't belong to a gym, not to worry—there are many exercises you can do at home that will give you the same results you would get at a gym, such as push-ups, wall-presses, and lunges. Following are some exercises to get you started, both at home and at the gym. And don't forget—every little bit counts, so make the most of every day, log your time (there's a spot in your Food Log to keep track of exercise), and see how it adds up by the end of the week!

Strength Training at Home

Push-Ups (for the chest, shoulders, and back): Place hands on floor, shoulder-width apart. Place your feet (toes pointed toward the floor) behind you so that your body is straight. Bend your elbows and lower your chest to the floor. Then push your body up off the ground by extending your arms. Repeat. (For an easier version, bend your knees and support your body weight with your hands and knees rather than with your hands and toes.) Note: Be sure your head is aligned with your body and is not sagging.

Wall Push-Down (for the chest): Place your hands against a wall shoulder-width apart. Stand about a foot away from the wall and push with your hands as hard as you can, as if you were trying to knock down the wall. Hold for 30 seconds and repeat.

Superman (for the lower back): Lie flat on your stomach with your arms extended above your head. Lift your right arm and left leg as high as you can off the ground at the same time and hold for 10 seconds. Repeat with left arm and right leg.

Biceps Curls (for biceps): Hold a weight in each hand and stand up straight with your body aligned, head facing forward. With arms by your sides, palms facing forward, slowly curl your forearms up toward your shoulders by bending your elbows. Release slowly and repeat. Note: Keep your wrists straight and your body still.

Dumbbell Kick Back (for triceps): Stand upright with your feet shoulder-width apart, holding a weight in each hand. Keeping your back straight, bend forward at the waist so your torso is about 45 degrees from upright. Keeping your upper arms at your sides, bring the dumbbells forward, bending your elbows at a 90-degree angle. Slowly extend the dumbbells back, straightening your arms behind you. Slowly return to starting position and repeat.

Frontal Lunge (for legs and butt): Stand with your feet shoulder-width apart, abs tight, and hands on hips. Lunge forward with one leg, keeping your torso upright, knees bent at 90 degrees, and thigh parallel to the floor. Make sure your knee does not go farther forward than your toe. Return to start and repeat with the other leg.

Dog at Hydrant (for glutes, hamstrings, and outer thighs): On a mat, get down on your hands and knees with your toes pointing toward the floor. Keep your back straight and your head aligned with your spine. Keeping your knee bent at a 90-degree angle, lift one leg up and out to the side until your thigh is parallel to the floor. Hold for 2 seconds before lowering the leg back down to start position. Repeat with the other leg.

Plank (for abs): Lie face down on a mat, bending your arms at the elbow and resting your forearms on the mat beneath your shoulders. Push yourself up onto your toes and continue to rest your upper body on your forearms, keeping your back flat and your abs pulled in tight. Hold the position for 20–60 seconds, depending on your strength. Lower and repeat for 3 repetitions.

Reverse Crunch (for lower abs): Lie on your back with your arms resting on the floor at your sides and your legs slightly bent and lifted off the floor, thighs aligned over your hips. Contract your abs and slowly roll your knees in toward your chin; with control, lower to starting position. Do not use momentum to move your knees.

Strength Training at the Gym

Pec Deck (for chest): Adjust the seat of the pec deck machine so that your elbows are aligned with your shoulders. Sit with your torso erect against the backrest and place your forearms against the resistance pads. Contract your abdominals to stabilize your body and squeeze the resistance pads together in front of your chest. Contract your chest muscles hard at the top of the movement and slowly return to starting position. Repeat.

Lat Pull-Down (for back): Adjust the seat of the pull-down machine so that your knees are bent comfortably under the thigh pad. Grasp the cable bar slightly wider than shoulder width with your palms facing the weight stack. Keeping your abdomen contracted, lean back 30 degrees from your hips. Squeeze your back muscles together as you pull the bar down toward your chest. Pause and then return to extended position. Repeat.

Shoulder Dumbbell Press (for shoulders): Sit on an upright bench with a dumbbell in each hand. Contract your abs and, with your palms facing forward, lift both dumbbells into the air so that each dumbbell is about level with your chin. Using your shoulders, press each dumbbell straight up overhead until they lightly touch. Pause, then slowly lower your arms back down to where both elbows are at a right angle, just about shoulder height. Repeat.

Machine Biceps Curl (for biceps): Sit on a bicep machine with your back flush against the back pad. Adjust your arms so that the back of your arms rest comfortably on the pad. Make sure your arms rest against the pad at all times. Relax your elbows, keep your wrists neutral, and grasp the bar with your hands shoulder-width apart. While contracting your biceps, raise the bar to the top position. Slowly lower the bar, stopping just before your elbows are straight, and repeat.

Triceps Press-Down (for triceps): Stand in front of a high cable machine with your feet shoulder-width apart. Add a V-bar attachment and grab it with your palms facing the floor. Keep your elbows at your sides and draw your navel inward. Press the V-bar down with your hands. As you pass the 90-degree elbow position, straighten your arms down and squeeze your triceps hard. Slowly bring the V-bar back up until your elbows are at a 90-degree angle. Repeat.

Leg Extension (for quadriceps): Sit on a leg extension machine and hook your feet behind the pad. Adjust the machine so that it is comfortable and the leg extension arm is right below your shinbone. Slowly contract your quadriceps and straighten your legs, pushing the weight up. Pause, then slowly lower your legs until just before your knees are straight. Pause and repeat.

Horizontal Leg Press (for hamstrings and butt): Sit on the leg press machine with your feet shoulder-width apart. Hold the handles and contract your abdominals. Keeping your knees over your ankles and your entire foot in contact with the foot plate, bend your knees to a 90-degree angle. Without locking your knees, straighten your legs. Slowly return to starting position and repeat.

Hip Adductor (for inner thighs): Sit with your back pressed into the adductor machine and your hands gripping the handles. Press the inside of your thighs against the resistance pads with your feet firmly on the footrests. Your legs should be spread apart as far as is comfortable.

Contract your inner thigh muscles and press your knees against the resistance pads to slowly and smoothly bring your thighs together. Hold for 2 seconds, then slowly return to a starting position, without letting the weight stack touch. Repeat.

Hip Abductor (for outer thighs): Sit with your back pressed into the abductor machine and your hands gripping the handles. Press the outside of your thighs against the resistance pads with your feet firmly on the footrests. Your legs should be as close together as possible. Contract your outer thigh muscles and press your knees against the resistance pads to slowly and smoothly bring your thighs out to the sides as far as they will go. Hold for 2 seconds, then slowly return to a starting position, without letting the weight stack touch. Repeat.

Following our Jumpstart and Maintenance plans and combining them with our cardio and weightlifting regimen will aid in your body transformation—morphing your body into a lean, toned, and sculpted body that everyone will envy. You will be fueling your body with wholesome, nutrient-rich foods and will be amazed by your energy that makes exercising easy—and most of all, you'll be in awe of your sculpted body. The recipes in the next chapter will help you make your slimming process even more enjoyable, as the recipes are absolutely delicious!

Chapter 10

The Nutrition Twins Favorite Skinny Recipes

In this chapter, you'll find our favorite delicious low-sodium recipes. You'll notice that some of them do include salt; however, the amount added is minimal so the total sodium in the meal remains low. Also, you may notice in some recipes that not every ingredient would be found on the Jumpstart Plan lists; however, like the added salt, these ingredients are added in small enough quantities to allow for a healthy overall recipe. For a recipe to qualify for the Jumpstart Plan, it must not contain more than 100 milligrams of sodium above the number of calories it contains. So, for example, for a recipe that has 268 calories, it must have 368 milligrams of sodium or less to be permitted on the Jumpstart Plan. All of the recipes (with the exception of just a few and some of the desserts) are so healthy that they can be used at any time— whether you are in the Jumpstart Phase or the Maintenance Phase. The few recipes that can't be used during the Jumpstart Phase are still very healthy and can be used during the Maintenance Phase and are noted as such. Enjoy!

Contents

Almond-Crusted Shrimp

⚛

½ cup ground almonds

3 tablespoons all-purpose flour

1 teaspoon minced fresh parsley *(or ½ teaspoon dried parsley)*

½ teaspoon seafood seasoning *(like Mrs. Dash Lemon Pepper seasoning blend)*

¼ teaspoon salt

¼ teaspoon black pepper

1 pound shrimp *(61- to 70-count)*, shelled and deveined, tails removed

1 egg white

2 tablespoons almond or corn oil, divided

1 lemon, cut into wedges

Stir together almonds, flour, parsley, seafood seasoning, salt, and pepper. Dip each shrimp in egg white, then in almond mixture; lay on a baking sheet or platter until ready to cook. Heat 1 tablespoon oil in a large skillet; cook shrimp in batches over medium heat for 3 to 4 minutes, turning once, until pink and golden. Use remaining 1 tablespoon oil as necessary. Serve shrimp immediately, accompanied by lemon wedges.

Nutrition Facts Per Serving: Makes 4 servings; Calories 316, Total Fat 15 grams, Saturated Fat 1.6 grams, Carbohydrates 17 grams, Protein 28 grams, Fiber 2 grams, Sodium 329 milligrams Count as: ½ Carbohydrate Slimmer, 1½ Protein Slimmers, 1 Mono Slimmer

From www.AlmondBoard.com

Asian Steak with Grapes

∽

12 ounces beef flank steak

2 tablespoons reduced-sodium soy sauce

2 tablespoons dry white wine

1 clove garlic, minced

1 teaspoon sesame oil

½ teaspoon crushed red chilies

½ cup sliced onion

1¼ cups halved California seedless grapes

¾ cup sliced sweet red pepper

2 tablespoons chopped green onions

1¾ cups finely shredded cabbage

1 teaspoon toasted sesame seeds

Slice steak into thin strips, cutting across the grain, and place in small bowl. Mix soy sauce, wine, garlic, sesame oil, and chilies in small bowl; stir well. Pour sauce over beef. Coat all pieces, cover, and marinate 20 minutes.

Place marinated beef and onion in a 2-quart microwave-safe dish. Cover with waxed paper. Microwave on high 4 minutes, stirring halfway through cooking. Add grapes, red pepper, and green onions; microwave on high 1 minute; mix well.

Place hot beef mixture on a bed of cabbage. Sprinkle with sesame seeds and serve.

Nutrition Facts Per Serving: Makes 4 servings; Calories 212, Total Fat 8 grams, Saturated Fat 3 grams, Protein 20 grams, Carbohydrates 13 grams, Fiber 2 grams, Sodium 316 milligrams
Count as: 2 Protein Slimmers, ¾ Flushers/Anti-Bloaters

Avocado and Grapefruit Chicken

ℰ

4 boneless chicken breasts halves

Paprika and white pepper, to season

1 teaspoon olive oil

1 cup reduced-sodium, fat-free chicken broth

1 cup grapefruit juice

2 tablespoons honey

1 medium onion, sliced

1½ large cloves garlic, minced

1 cup dry orzo *(rice-shaped pasta)* or 3 cups of cooked rice

½ teaspoon cornstarch

2 teaspoons each fresh tarragon and thyme leaves

1 ripe fresh California avocado, seeded, peeled, and sliced

1 large grapefruit, peeled and sectioned

Remove any excess fat from chicken; rinse and pat dry. Lightly sprinkle chicken with paprika and pepper.

In a large nonstick skillet sprayed with no-stick cooking spray, heat oil. Over medium-high heat, quickly brown chicken on both sides, about 5 minutes. Add ½ cup broth, grapefruit juice, honey, onion, and garlic; bring to a boil. Lower the heat; cover and simmer for 10 to 12 minutes, until chicken is tender.

Remove chicken and place on cooked orzo or rice; keep warm.

Mix cornstarch with remaining ½ cup broth; stir into skillet mixture. Add tarragon and thyme. Cook, stirring until sauce thickens. Add avocado and grapefruit; heat briefly. Serve sauce over chicken and brown rice.

Nutrition Facts Per Serving: Makes 6 servings; Calories 324, Total Fat 7 grams, Saturated Fat 1 gram, Carbohydrates 43 grams, Protein 21 grams, Fiber 2 grams, Sodium 146 milligrams Count as: 1½ Protein Slimmers, 1½ Carbohydrate Slimmers, ½ Mono Slimmer, ½ Flusher/Anti-Bloater

Baja Fish Tacos with Mango Salsa

∽

Mango Salsa:

2 large ripe mangos, peeled, pitted, and chopped into bite-size pieces

¼ cup minced red bell pepper

1 tablespoon lime juice

1 tablespoon chopped fresh cilantro

2 green onions, sliced *(green tops only)*

1 small jalapeño pepper, minced, stem, seeds, and membrane removed

Tacos:

1 pound cod fillets, rinsed and patted dry

1 teaspoon chili powder

½ teaspoon ground cumin

½ teaspoon Mexican oregano

½ teaspoon garlic salt

8 corn tortillas, warmed

2 cups shredded green or red cabbage

½ cup crumbled cotija cheese *(may substitute shredded low-fat Monterey Jack)*

Preheat oven to 425°F. Stir together mango, bell pepper, lime juice, cilantro, onions, and jalapeño in a medium bowl; set aside. Place cod on 2 large sheets of parchment paper. Stir together dry seasonings in a small bowl and sprinkle over cod. Bring edges of parchment paper together and fold twice. Fold ends under to enclose fish. Place packets on a baking sheet and bake for 15 to 18 minutes. Open packets carefully to let steam escape. Place equal amounts of cod in each tortilla and top with cabbage, cheese, and mango salsa.

Nutrition Facts Per Serving: Makes 4 Servings; Calories 337, Total Fat 8 grams, Saturated Fat 1½ grams, Carbohydrates 45 grams, Protein 29 grams, Fiber 7 grams, Sodium 285 milligrams Count as: 1 Carbohydrate Slimmer, 2 Protein Slimmers, 1 Flusher/Anti-Bloater

From The National Mango Board

Blazing Glory Raspberry Chicken Breasts

∾

This is an easy and tasty entrée. The seasoning and raspberry preserves supply the flavor punch for simple grilled chicken breasts.

½ cup water

⅓ cup white wine vinegar

2 tablespoons McCormick Grill Mates Roasted Garlic & Herb Seasoning

2 teaspoons cornstarch

½ cup raspberry preserves

2 pounds boneless skinless chicken breast halves

Mix the water, vinegar, McCormick seasoning, and cornstarch in small saucepan until cornstarch is completely dissolved. Bring to boil on medium heat, stirring constantly. Cook and stir about 4 minutes or until mixture thickens. Add preserves; stir until melted. Cool completely. Reserve ⅓ cup of the marinade for basting.

Place chicken in large resealable plastic bag or glass dish. Pour remaining marinade over chicken; turn to coat well. Refrigerate 30 minutes or longer for extra flavor. Remove chicken from marinade. Discard any remaining marinade.

Grill over medium heat 10 to 12 minutes or until cooked through, turning occasionally and basting with reserved marinade.

Nutrition Facts Per Serving: Makes 8 servings. Calories 162, Total Fat 2 grams, Saturated Fat ½ gram, Carbohydrates 15 grams, Protein 21 grams, Fiber 0, Sodium 242 milligrams
Count as: 2 Protein Slimmers

From www.mccormick.com

Caramelized Salmon with Tropical Salsa

Salmon, rich in omega-3 fatty acids, teams up with tropical fruits and cherries for a healthy, deliciously sweet, and savory entree.

1½ pounds fresh or frozen salmon fillet with skin

3 tablespoons brown sugar

1¼ tablespoons grated orange peel

½ teaspoon coarsely ground pepper

1 cup ripe mango or papaya, seeded, peeled, and chopped

1 cup frozen tart cherries, thawed, drained, and halved

2 tablespoons chopped fresh mint

2 teaspoons balsamic vinegar

¼ teaspoon crushed red pepper

Stir together brown sugar, orange peel, and pepper. Place fish, skin side down, in a shallow pan. Rub sugar mixture over fish. Cover and refrigerate 2 to 8 hours. Remove fish from pan, draining juices. Place salmon, skin-side down, on gas grill over medium heat. Grill for 20 to 25 minutes, or until fish flakes easily. Do not turn fish. Meanwhile, toss together mango or papaya, cherries, mint, vinegar, and red pepper. Spoon fruit salsa over warm fish. Serve immediately.

Nutrition Facts Per Serving: Makes 4 servings; Calories 350, Total Fat 13 grams, Saturated Fat 3 grams, Carbohydrates 24 grams, Protein 37 grams, Fiber 2 grams, Sodium 93 milligrams Count as: 2½ Protein Slimmers, 1 Flusher/Anti-Bloater

Creamy Chicken Penne

∾

A light cream sauce with a delicious trio of Mediterranean herbs is tossed with penne, chicken, and broccoli. It has a decadent flavor that you can enjoy without the guilt.

8 ounces uncooked multigrain penne pasta

1½ cups fresh or frozen broccoli florets

1 cup fat-free half-and-half

4 ounces Neufchâtel cheese, cubed

1 teaspoon McCormick Oregano Leaves

1 teaspoon McCormick Rosemary Leaves, finely crushed

1 teaspoon McCormick Thyme Leaves

½ teaspoon McCormick Garlic Powder

¼ teaspoon Sea Salt from McCormick Sea Salt Grinder

1½ cups chopped cooked chicken breast

2 tablespoons grated Parmesan or Asiago cheese

Cook pasta in large saucepan as directed on package, adding broccoli during the last 3 minutes of cooking. Drain well.

Meanwhile, bring half-and-half to simmer in small saucepan on medium heat. Reduce heat to medium-low. Add Neufchâtel cheese, oregano, rosemary, thyme, garlic powder, and sea salt; whisk until cheese is melted and sauce is well blended. Add chicken; simmer until heated through.

Place pasta and broccoli in a large serving bowl. Spoon sauce evenly over pasta mixture. Toss gently to coat well. Sprinkle with Parmesan cheese and serve immediately.

Nutrition Facts Per Serving: Makes 6 servings; Calories 283, Total Fat 7 grams. Saturated Fat 3 grams, Carbohydrates 32 grams, Protein 23 grams, Fiber 3 grams, Sodium 271 milligrams Count as: 1½ Carbohydrate Slimmers, 1½ Protein Slimmers, ½ Flusher/Anti-Bloater

From www.mccormick.com

Ginger Shrimp with Gai Lan

∽

Gai lan is known as Chinese broccoli or Chinese kale. If you can't find it, you can substitute broccoli or Swiss chard.

5 large dry shiitake mushrooms, soaked in water and sliced

2 tablespoons canola oil

½ pound large uncooked shrimp

1 medium onion, cut into wedges

1 clove garlic, minced

5 large stalks gai lan, cut into medium-sized pieces *(or broccoli or Swiss chard)*

1 tablespoon fresh ginger, minced

⅛ teaspoon five spice powder

1 tablespoon sweet chili sauce

1 tablespoon cornstarch

1 cup low-sodium chicken broth

¼ cup unsalted cashew nuts, coarsely chopped

Soak mushrooms in water for about 30 minutes.

Pour canola oil into large wok and heat over medium-high heat. Quickly stir-fry shrimp until just cooked. Remove from wok. Add a bit more canola oil if necessary. Add onion, garlic, gai lan stalks (leave out leafy parts until the end of cooking time), ginger, five spice powder and sweet chili sauce. Stir-fry for 3-4 minutes to cook vegetables. Dissolve cornstarch in broth and add to vegetables. Heat mixture for 1 minute.

Add shrimp and gai lan leaves to the mixture and heat through. Garnish with cashew nuts and serve immediately.

Nutrition Facts Per Serving: Makes 4 servings; Calories 90, Total Fat 3.5 grams, Saturated Fat 0, Carbohydrates 13 grams, Protein 10 grams, Fiber 0, Sodium 60 milligrams
Count as: 1 Protein Slimmer, ⅙ Mono Slimmer

From www.canolainfo.org

Grilled Lemon Pepper Herb Salmon

Delicious salmon is easy with Grill Mates Lemon Pepper with Herbs. Serve with Cucumber Sour Cream Sauce, if desired.

1 tablespoon olive oil

1½ pounds salmon fillets

2 teaspoons McCormick Grill Mates Lemon Pepper with Herbs Seasoning

Cucumber Sour Cream Sauce:

6 ounces plain, low-fat yogurt

½ cup low-fat sour cream

½ cup finely chopped, peeled, and seeded cucumber

2 tablespoons chopped fresh parsley

1 teaspoon Grill Mates Lemon Pepper with Herbs

Rub oil over flesh side of fish; sprinkle evenly with Seasoning. Grill over medium-high heat 6 to 7 minutes per side or until fish flakes easily with a fork. Serve with Cucumber Sour Cream Sauce, if desired.

For Sour Cream Sauce: Mix yogurt, low-fat sour cream, 1 cucumber, parsley, and Grill Mates Lemon Pepper with Herbs seasoning in small bowl; cover. Refrigerate until ready to serve. Spoon about 2 tablespoons sauce over each salmon fillet. Refrigerate any leftover sauce. Makes 1¼ cups.

Nutrition Facts Per Serving: Makes 6 servings; Calories 168, Total Fat 8 grams, Saturated Fat 3 grams, Carbohydrates 0, Protein 24 grams, Fiber 0, Sodium 170 milligrams
Count as: 2½ Protein Slimmers, 1 Anti-Bloater/Flusher

From www.mccormick.com

Grilled Lemon-Pepper Herb Shrimp Kabobs on Brown Rice

✑

1 pound large shrimp, peeled and deveined

1 tablespoon olive oil

2 teaspoons McCormick Grill Mates Lemon Pepper with Herbs Seasoning

4 cups assorted fresh vegetable pieces, such as mushrooms, squash, onion, and zucchini

2 cups brown rice

Toss shrimp with oil in large resealable plastic bag or glass bowl. Add seasoning; toss again until shrimp are evenly coated. Alternately thread shrimp and vegetables onto metal skewers.

Grill over medium heat 8 to 10 minutes or until shrimp turn pink and vegetables are tender, turning frequently. Serve over ½ cup steamed brown rice.

Nutrition Facts Per Serving: Makes 4 servings; Calories 261, Total Fat 6 grams, Saturated Fat ½ gram, Carbohydrates 29 grams, Protein 22 grams, Fiber 4 grams, Sodium 369 milligrams Count as: 1½ Protein Slimmers, 1 Carbohydrate Slimmer, 1 Flusher/Anti-Bloater

From www.mccormick.com

Herbed Salmon Burgers

∽

Use in Maintenance Phase Only

Sauce:

½ cup plain nonfat yogurt

⅓ cup seeded, chopped tomato

⅓ cup seeded, chopped cucumber

1½ tablespoons finely chopped onion

¾ tablespoon finely chopped fresh dill or 1 teaspoon dried dill weed

Salmon Cakes:

1 14¾-ounce can pink salmon, drained, skin and bones removed

¾ cup Quaker Oats *(quick or old-fashioned, uncooked)*

⅓ cup fat-free milk

2 egg whites, lightly beaten

1 tablespoon finely chopped onion

1 tablespoon finely chopped fresh dill or 1 teaspoon dried dill weed

Mix the yogurt, tomato, cucumber, onion, and dill in small bowl. Cover and chill while making salmon cakes.

Combine all ingredients for salmon cakes in medium bowl; mix well. Let stand 5 minutes. Make 5 oval patties about 1 inch thick.

Lightly spray non-stick skillet with non-stick cooking spray. Cook salmon cakes over medium heat, 3 to 4 minutes on each side, or until golden brown and heated through. Serve with sauce.

Nutrition Facts Per Serving: Makes 5 servings; Calories 170, Fat 6 grams, Saturated Fat 1 gram, Carbohydrates 12 grams, Protein 19 grams, Fiber 2 grams, Sodium 400 milligrams
Count as: ½ Carbohydrate Slimmer, 1½ Protein Slimmers

Peppery Tuna

⤫

½ cup plain nonfat yogurt

½ tablespoon olive oil

4 five-ounce tuna steaks

juice and zest from one lemon

1½ tablespoons cracked black pepper

3 tablespoons chopped parsley

1 pound fresh spinach leaves

Salt to taste *(Use cautiously!)*

Combine yogurt and oil. Brush the tuna steaks with the yogurt mixture. Combine lemon zest (reserve juice), pepper, and parsley and sprinkle onto tuna steaks. Let stand 20 minutes.

Preheat grill. Lightly salt tuna and grill 3-4 minutes per side. Meanwhile, steam spinach; season as desired and sprinkle with lemon juice. Divide among four plates and top with tuna steak.

Nutrition Facts Per Serving: Makes 4 servings; Calories 200, Total Fat 3.5 grams, Saturated Fat 1 gram, Carbohydrates 9 grams, Protein 36 grams, Fiber 4 grams, Sodium 170 milligrams
Count as: 2 Protein Slimmers, 1½ Flushers/Anti-Bloaters

Peruvian Ceviche with Potatoes, Halibut, and Mango

∽

1 pound white potatoes, peeled, and cut into ¼-inch cubes

1 cup fresh or frozen corn kernels

1 pound skinned halibut, black bass, striped bass, or tile
fish, cut into ½-inch pieces

1 large mango, peeled, seeded, and chopped

½ cup halved, thinly sliced red onion

1 small fresh jalapeño chile, stemmed, seeded, and minced

½ cup fresh lime juice

¼ cup minced cilantro

½ teaspoon salt

½ teaspoon freshly ground black pepper

6 large lettuce leaves

Bring a large saucepan of water to a boil over high heat. Add the potatoes; boil for 5 minutes.

Add the corn and boil until the potatoes are tender, about 5 minutes. Drain in a colander set in the sink, place in a large nonreactive bowl (see note below), and cool to room temperature, about 1 hour.

Add the fish, mango, onion, jalapeño, lime juice, cilantro, salt, and pepper; toss well. Cover and refrigerate for at least 6 hours or up to 24 hours, tossing occasionally. Serve in lettuce cups.

Note: A nonreactive bowl is one that will not form harmful chemical compounds when acid (as in the lime juice here) touches its surface. Nonreactive materials include heat-safe glass, stainless steel, enameled iron, or enameled steel. Reactive cookware is made of tin, copper, and non-anodized aluminum; certain dyes and chemicals in decorative glass and pottery are also reactive.

Nutrition Facts Per Serving: Makes 6 servings; Calories 198, Total Fat 2 grams, Saturated Fat 0, Carbohydrates 27 grams, Protein 19 grams, Fiber 3 grams, Sodium 245 milligrams
Count as: 1 Carbohydrate Slimmer, 1 Protein Slimmer

From www.potatogoodness.com

Pesto Deviled Eggs

ᥴᡐ

With high-quality protein and less than 100 calories each, deviled eggs make a great snack.

6 hard-cooked eggs
3 tablespoons grated Parmesan cheese
2 tablespoons plain low-fat yogurt
1 teaspoon basil leaves, crushed
½ teaspoon garlic powder

Cut eggs in half lengthwise. Remove yolks and set whites aside. Mash yolks with fork. Stir in remaining ingredients until well blended. Refill whites, using about 1 tablespoon yolk mixture for each egg half. Chill to blend flavors.

Nutrition Facts Per Serving of ⅙ **recipe:** Makes 6 servings; Calories 93, Total Fat 6 grams, Carbohydrates 1 gram, Protein 8 grams, Fiber 0, Sodium 112 milligrams
Count as: 1 Protein Slimmer

From www.IncredibleEgg.org

The Nutrition Twins Skinny Bean and Veggie Tostitos

இ

1 teaspoon olive oil

1 cup diced onion

¾ cup diced red bell pepper

¾ cup diced green bell pepper

¼ cup chopped zucchini

1 tablespoon chili powder

2 teaspoons dried oregano

1 teaspoon ground cumin

1 garlic clove, minced

1 cup canned chickpeas *(garbanzo beans)*, rinsed and drained *(Or try this "salternative": canned Eden Organic Garbanzo Beans No Salt Added or raw garbanzos, boiled and drained)*

½ cup canned black beans, rinsed and drained *(Or try this "salternative": Eden Organic Black Beans, No Salt Added or raw black beans, boiled and drained)*

½ cup canned pinto beans, rinsed and drained *(Or try this "salternative": Eden Organic Pinto Beans, No Salt Added or raw pinto beans, boiled and drained)*

1 8-ounce can No Salt Added tomato sauce

Tostitos, 1 large bag *(use 5-6 chips for scooping per serving)*

¾ cup shredded iceberg or romaine lettuce

¾ cup diced tomato

½ cup finely shredded reduced-fat cheddar or Monterey Jack cheese

½ cup low-sodium or no-salt-added salsa, like Enrico's No Salt Added Chunky Salsa

Heat oil in a large nonstick skillet over medium-high heat until hot.

Add onion and next 7 ingredients (onion through garlic), and sauté 2 minutes. Add chickpeas, beans, and tomato sauce.

Bring to a boil; reduce heat, and simmer 20 minutes or until thick.

Spoon ¼ cup bean mixture onto the Tostitos.

Top each serving with lettuce, 1 tablespoon tomato, 2 teaspoons cheese, and 2 teaspoons salsa.

Nutrition Facts Per Serving: Makes 12 servings; Calories 152, Total Fat 6 grams, Saturated Fat 1 gram, Carbohydrates 21 grams, Protein 6 grams, Fiber 4 grams, Sodium 216 milligrams
Count as: 1 Carbohydrate Slimmer, ¼ Protein Slimmer, 1 Flusher/Anti-Bloater

The Nutrition Twins Skinny Chicken Parm

∽

4 3-ounce skinless chicken breasts

4 egg whites

⅔ cup unseasoned bread crumbs *(Or for a healthy, improved "salternative," blend 2 slices whole-grain bread to use as bread crumbs)*

¾ cup low-fat shredded cheese

4 tablespoons fat-free Parmesan cheese

2 cups Walnut Acres Low-Sodium Tomato and Basil Pasta sauce *(or other low-sodium tomato sauce with less than 40 calories per serving)*

garlic powder, to taste

pepper, to taste

Rinse the chicken breast with water.

Preheat oven to 350°F. Dip the chicken in egg whites (or just use the water from cleaning to stick the breading).

Pour bread crumbs into a plastic bag. Toss chicken in one piece at a time, shaking bag to cover the chicken with the breading.

Shake off excess breading. Put the chicken in a shallow glass dish and bake for approximately 25 minutes until chicken is thoroughly cooked.

When chicken is done, cover with cheese and sprinkle with the Parmesan cheese.

Put it back in the oven until the cheese has melted. While the cheese is melting, heat marinara sauce on the stove or in the microwave.

When the cheese is melted, take the chicken out of the oven and place on plates. Pour the heated sauce on top. Serve and enjoy!

Nutrition Facts Per Serving: Makes 4 servings; Calories 291, Total Fat 8 grams, Saturated Fat 4 grams, Carbohydrates 18 grams, Protein 35 grams, Dietary Fiber 1 gram, Sodium 391 milligrams Count as: 2 Protein Slimmers, ½ Carb Slimmer, 1 Flusher/Anti-Bloater

The Nutrition Twins Skinny Hawaiian Chicken

∾

The pineapple adds a delicious sweetness to the chicken, not to mention a boost of vitamin C.

1 8-ounce can unsweetened pineapple slices, packed in juice

1 teaspoon chopped garlic

1 teaspoon cornstarch

1 bell pepper

1 medium onion

1 teaspoon Worcestershire sauce

1 teaspoon Dijon mustard

½ teaspoon dried thyme

⅛ teaspoon ginger

4 skinless, boneless chicken breasts *(about 1 pound)*

Preheat oven to 400°F.

Wash bell pepper and cut into bite-sized pieces. Peel and slice onion and set aside with peppers. Drain pineapple, saving the juice.

Combine the pineapple juice with garlic, cornstarch, Worcestershire, mustard, thyme, and ginger.

Spray an 8" x 8" baking pan with non-stick cooking spray. Place the chicken in the pan and top with the peppers and onions. Pour the juice mixture over the chicken and vegetables.

Bake for 20 minutes. Spoon juices from pan over chicken. Add a pineapple slice to each piece of chicken and heat for another 5 minutes or until chicken is thoroughly cooked.

Nutrition Facts Per Serving: Makes 4 servings; Calories 170, Total Fat 3 grams, Saturated Fat ½ gram, Carbohydrates 10 grams, Protein 26 grams, Fiber 3 grams, Sodium 101 milligrams
Count as: 1¾ Protein Slimmers, 1 Flusher/Anti-Bloater

The Nutrition Twins Skinny Rosemary Turkey with Vegetables

⌒

1 pound turkey breast tenderloin slices, all visible fat removed
½ cup low-sodium chicken broth
1 tablespoon cornstarch
⅛ teaspoon salt
⅛ teaspoon black pepper
vegetable oil spray
2 tablespoons balsamic vinegar
1 teaspoon snipped fresh rosemary or ¼ teaspoon dried rosemary, crushed
10 ounces chanterelle or button mushrooms, cleaned, trimmed, and sliced
2 carrots, peeled and sliced
2 celery stalks, sliced
¼ cup chopped shallots or onion
Fresh rosemary *(optional)*

Rinse turkey, pat dry, and set aside.

In a small bowl, stir together broth, cornstarch, salt, and pepper. Set aside.

Spray a large skillet with vegetable oil and place over medium-high heat.

Add half the turkey to hot skillet. Cook about 2 minutes per side, or until turkey is tender and no longer pink. Repeat with remaining turkey.

Move skillet away from heat. Remove turkey from skillet and keep warm.

Add vinegar and rosemary to skillet, stirring to scrape up brown bits from bottom of pan. Return skillet to heat, and add mushrooms, carrots, celery, and shallots or onion.

Over medium heat, cook and stir until vegetables are tender, about 8 minutes. Stir broth mixture and add to skillet. Cook and stir until thickened and bubbly, approximately 3 minutes. Cook 2 minutes more, stirring constantly. Serve sauce with turkey. Serve on a bed of rosemary, if desired.

Nutrition Facts Per Serving (with 2 tablespoons of sauce per serving): Makes 4 servings; Calories 169, Total Fat 4 grams, Saturated Fat 1 gram, Carbohydrates 5 grams, Protein 28 grams, Fiber 2.5 grams, Sodium 137 milligrams
Count as: 1¾ Protein Slimmers, 1 Flusher/Anti-Bloater

The Nutrition Twins Summertime Salsa Chicken

cℐↄ

1 cucumber, peeled and diced

1 tomato, diced

½ red onion, diced

1 red pepper, diced

1 red apple, peeled and diced

juice from 2 limes

6 4-ounce chicken breasts

In mixing bowl, stir all ingredients (except for the chicken) together. Then refrigerate.

Grill chicken over medium flame until cooked through. Pour cold salsa on hot chicken and serve.

Nutrition Facts Per Serving: Makes 6 servings; Calories 217, Total Fat 4 grams, Saturated Fat 1 gram, Carbohydrates 9 grams, Protein 35 grams, Fiber 2 grams, Sodium 86 milligrams
Count as: 2 Protein Slimmers, ½ Flusher

White Bean and Rosemary Chicken

⌒∅

We love Italian food like this. It's ready in 30 minutes.

⅓ cup Italian dressing (preferably low-sodium)

4 boneless, skinless chicken breasts *(about 1¼ pounds)*

¼ cup water

3 medium carrots, sliced *(1½ cups)*

3 medium stalks celery, sliced *(1½ cups)*

¼ cup coarsely chopped drained sun-dried tomatoes in oil

1 teaspoon dried rosemary leaves, crushed

1 can *(19-ounce)* cannellini beans, drained and rinsed

Heat the dressing over medium-high heat in a 12-inch skillet. Cook chicken in dressing 2 to 3 minutes on each side or until lightly browned.

Lower heat to medium-low. Add water, carrots, celery, tomatoes, and rosemary to skillet.

Cover and simmer about 10 minutes or until carrots are crisp-tender and juice of chicken is clear when center of thickest part is cut (170°F).

Stir in beans. Cover; cook 5 to 6 minutes or until beans are thoroughly heated.

Check chicken for doneness at the minimum cooking time by cutting into the thickest part of the chicken with a knife to see if the juices are clear.

Nutrition Facts Per Serving: Makes 4 servings; Calories 392, Total Fat 9 grams, Saturated Fat 2 grams, Carbohydrates 33 grams, Protein 42 grams, Fiber 9 grams, Sodium 340 milligrams Count as: 2 Protein Slimmers, 1¼ Carbohydrate Slimmers, 1 Condiment Slimmer, ½ Flusher/ Anti-Bloater

Zucchini Lasagna

⁓

½ pound cooked lasagna noodles, cooked in unsalted water
¾ cup part-skim mozzarella cheese, grated
1½ cups fat-free cottage cheese*
¼ cup Parmesan cheese, grated
1½ cups raw zucchini, sliced
2½ cups low-sodium tomato sauce
2 teaspoons basil, dried
2 teaspoons oregano, dried
¼ cup onion, chopped
1 clove garlic
⅛ teaspoon black pepper

Preheat oven to 350°F. Lightly spray a 9 x 13-inch baking dish with vegetable oil spray.

In a small bowl, combine ⅛ cup mozzarella and 1 tablespoon Parmesan cheese. Set aside.

In a medium bowl, combine remaining mozzarella and Parmesan cheese with all the cottage cheese. Mix well and set aside.

Combine tomato sauce with remaining ingredients. Spread a thin layer of tomato sauce in the bottom of the baking dish. Add a third of the noodles in a single layer. Spread half of the cottage cheese mixture on top. Add a layer of zucchini. Repeat layering. Add a thin coating of sauce. Top with noodles, sauce, and reserved cheese mixture. Cover with aluminum foil. Bake 30 to 40 minutes. Cool for 10 to 15 minutes. Cut into 6 portions.

Nutrition Facts Per Serving: Makes 6 servings; Calories 200, Total Fat 5 grams, Saturated Fat 3 grams, Carbohydrates 24 grams, Protein 15 grams, Fiber 3 grams, Sodium 368 milligrams
To reduce sodium, use low-sodium cottage cheese. New sodium content for each serving is 165 milligrams.
Count as: 1 Carbohydrate Slimmer, 1 Protein Slimmer, ½ Flusher/Anti-Bloater

From The National Heart, Lung, and Blood Institute

Nutrition Twins Skinny & Quick Peanut Bars

∽

1 cup unsalted peanuts

1 tablespoon minced fresh ginger

2 tablespoons sesame seeds

½ cup raisins

½ cup dates

2 tablespoons honey

Blend all ingredients (except for the honey) in a food processor until fairly smooth. Don't grind completely as you want some texture. Add the honey and blend just long enough for it to be incorporated.

On a plate or in a square pan, press the mixture into a square about ¾-inch thick and refrigerate for at least an hour. Cut into 2-inch squares.

Nutrition Facts Per 1-Bar Serving: Makes 8–10 bars; Calories 120, Total Fat 6 grams, Saturated Fat .5 gram, Carbohydrates 15 grams, Protein 4 grams, Fiber 2 grams, Sodium 3 milligrams Count as: 1 Mono Slimmer, ¼ Protein Slimmer

Nutrition Twins Skinny Peanut Butter Banana Roll-Up

∽

While the combination might sound strange, it is quick and delicious, too. This also makes a great breakfast on the run.

1 medium-sized banana

1 tablespoon all-natural peanut butter

1 slice whole-wheat bread like Pepperidge Farm's 100% Stoneground Whole Wheat Bread, or any other bread on the Jumpstart Carbohydrate Slimmers List

Spread peanut butter on the banana. Roll bread around banana and enjoy!

Nutrition Facts Per Serving: Calories 273, Total Fat 9 grams, Saturated Fat 2 grams, Carbohydrates 46 grams, Protein 7 grams, Fiber 7 grams, Sodium 129 milligrams
Count as: 1 Carbohydrate Slimmer, 1 Mono Slimmer, 1 Anti-Bloater/Flusher

Peach and Cream Pops

∽

½ cup peeled, chopped fresh California peaches

⅓ cup peeled, pureed fresh California peaches

⅔ cup nonfat vanilla yogurt

Lightly swirl all ingredients together in a small bowl. Spoon into 4 Popsicle molds and insert handle. Freeze for at least 4 hours.

Nutrition Facts Per Serving (1 Pop): Makes 4 pops; Calories 40, Total Fat 0, Saturated Fat 0, Carbohydrates 7 grams, Protein 2 grams, Fiber 1 gram, Sodium 25 milligrams
Count 1 Pop as: ¼ Anti-Bloater/Flusher, ¼ Protein Slimmer

From California Tree Fruit Agreement (CTFA)

PlumSmart Plum Berry Smoothie

✑

1 cup Sunsweet PlumSmart juice

1 cup frozen blueberries

½ cup fat-free plain yogurt

1 to 2 tablespoons honey

1 cup ice cubes

Puree all ingredients in a blender until smooth, adding more ice cubes if you prefer a thicker smoothie.

Nutrition Facts Per Serving (with blueberries): Makes 2 servings; Calories 190, Fat .5 gram, Saturated Fat 0, Carbohydrates 44 grams, Protein 3 grams, Fiber 3.5 grams, Sodium 63 milligrams Count as: 1½ Flushers/Anti-Bloaters and ½ Protein Slimmer

From Sunsweet Growers, Inc.

Spiced Orchard Popcorn Mix

∽

1½ teaspoons sugar

½ teaspoon apple pie spice blend

1 package 100-calorie microwave popcorn

⅓ cup dried tart cherries

⅓ cup dried blueberries

Butter-flavored non-stick cooking spray

Stir together sugar and apple pie spice in small bowl; set aside. Make popcorn according to the package directions and add the cherries and blueberries. Lightly spray with non-stick cooking spray. Sprinkle with sugar mixture; toss until coated.

Cinnamon-Spiced Orchard Popcorn: Prepare Spiced Orchard Popcorn as directed, except substitute ½ teaspoon ground cinnamon for the apple pie spice blend.

Red Hot Spiced Orchard Popcorn: Prepare Spiced Orchard Popcorn mix as directed, except substitute ¼ teaspoon ground allspice for the ½ teaspoon apple pie spice blend and season to taste with ground (cayenne) red pepper.

Nutrition Facts Per 2-Cup Serving: Makes about 2 (2-cup) servings; Calories 220, Total Fat 1 gram, Saturated Fat 0, Carbohydrates 47 grams, Protein 4 grams, Fiber 4 grams, Sodium 66 milligrams
Orchard Cinnamon-Spiced Popcorn: Nutrition Facts Per 2-Cup Serving: Calories 223, Total Fat 1 gram, Saturated Fat 0, Carbohydrates 47 grams, Protein 4 grams, Fiber 4 grams, Sodium 65 milligrams
Red Hot Spiced Orchard Popcorn: Nutrition Facts Per 2-Cup Serving: Calories 223, Total Fat 1 gram, Saturated Fat 0, Carbohydrates 47 grams, Protein 4 grams, Fiber 4 grams, Sodium 66 milligrams
Count as: 2 Carbohydrate Slimmers

Blueberry Protein Pancakes

೧෨

These make a great breakfast because they pack fruit, whole grains, and protein into a delicious pancake. They give you nutrients and long-lasting energy. Enjoy!

1 cup low-fat cottage cheese

¾ cup egg substitute *(equal to 3 eggs)*

¼ cup skim or fat-free milk

1 cup whole-wheat flour

2 tablespoons sugar or the equivalent in artificial sweetener
 (or 2 tablespoons of most artificial sweeteners)

1 cup blueberries

Combine the cottage cheese, egg substitute, milk, and flour in blender. Blend until smooth. Add the sugar and blend again.

Spray a pan with non-stick cooking spray. When hot, pour batter onto pan to make 12 pancakes. (If pan is small, you may have to cook in batches.) Sprinkle each pancake with blueberries. Cook until golden brown on both sides.

The blueberries add so much great flavor that these taste delicious without a topping. If you do want to add something, try sugar-free syrup, which will save you hundreds of calories over the regular version.

Nutrition Facts Per Serving (1 serving equals 2 pancakes): Makes 12 4-inch pancakes; Calories 125 (129 calories without artificial sweetener), Total Fat 1 gram, Saturated Fat 0, Carbohydrates 25 grams (20 grams with artificial sweetener), Protein 11 grams, Fiber 4 grams, Sodium 215 milligrams Count as: ¼ Carbohydrate Slimmer, ¾ Protein Slimmer, ½ Flusher

Cinnamon Orange French Toast

༂

Orange juice, vanilla, and nutmeg bring a surprising flavor to the French toast. You could also use apple cider with cinnamon bread or any other juice, flavoring, or spice you like, along with a different type of whole multi-grain bread.

6 eggs
1 tablespoon grated orange peel
½ cup orange juice
¼ cup nonfat or low-fat milk
⅓ cup sugar
½ teaspoon vanilla
¼ teaspoon ground nutmeg
8 slices day-old whole-grain raisin bread
Cooking spray
Confectioners' sugar *(optional)*
Orange slices *(optional)*

Preheat oven to 375°F.

In medium bowl, beat together eggs, orange peel, orange juice, milk, sugar, vanilla, and nutmeg until well blended.

Place bread in single layer in 13 x 9 x 2-inch pan. Pour egg mixture over bread. Let soak, turning once, until liquid is absorbed, about 5 minutes. Evenly coat 2 baking sheets with cooking spray. Place bread slices in single layer on sheets.

Bake for 12 to 15 minutes. Turn the slices over. Continue baking until browned, about 10 to 12 minutes.

Dust with confectioners' sugar and serve with orange slices, if desired. Just remember to count ½ orange as ½ Flusher/Anti-Bloater.

Nutrition Facts Per Serving: Makes 4 servings; *using 2% milk without optional ingredients:* Calories 332, Total Fat 9 grams, Saturated Fat 3 grams, Carbohydrates 49 grams, Protein 13 grams, Fiber 3 grams, Sodium 285 milligrams.
Count as: 2 Carbohydrate Slimmers, 1½ Protein Slimmers

From www.IncredibleEgg.org

Farmer's Market Omelet

⚙⁓

4 eggs

2 teaspoons grated Parmesan cheese

½ teaspoon basil leaves, crushed

¼ teaspoon garlic powder

Cooking spray

½ cup thinly sliced zucchini

½ cup thinly sliced yellow summer squash

½ cup sliced fresh mushrooms

¼ cup chopped sweet red pepper

¼ cup water, plus 2 additional tablespoons

In small saucepan over medium heat, sauté all of the vegetables with 2 tablespoons of water. Cover and cook just until vegetables are crisp-tender, about 3 to 4 minutes. Uncover and cook until liquid is evaporated. Cover and keep warm while preparing omelets.

In small bowl, beat together eggs, ¼ cup water, cheese, and seasonings until blended.

Spray a 7- to 10-inch nonstick skillet with cooking spray. Pour in ½ cup of the egg mixture so it sets immediately at edges.

With a spatula, carefully push cooked portions at edges toward center so uncooked portions can reach hot pan surface, tilting pan and moving cooked portions as necessary.

When top is thickened and no visible liquid egg remains, fill with half of the reserved vegetable mixture.

With pancake turner, fold omelet in half or roll. Invert onto plate with a quick flip of the wrist or slide from pan onto plate. Keep warm. Repeat with remaining egg and vegetable mixtures for second omelet.

Nutrition Facts Per Serving of ½ recipe using cooking spray: Makes 2 servings; Calories 180, Fat 11 grams, Saturated Fat 3 grams, Carbohydrates 5 grams, Protein 14 grams, Sodium 160 milligrams Count as: 2 Protein Slimmers, 1 Anti-Bloater/Flusher

From www.IncredibleEgg.org

The Nutrition Twins
StrawBluBanana Smoothie

cↄↄ

1 cup soy milk *(calcium-fortified)*

1 large banana

½ cup unsweetened fresh or frozen blueberries

½ cup unsweetened frozen strawberries

1 teaspoon dried flaxseed/linseed

Combine soy milk, banana, blueberries, strawberries, and flaxseed/linseed in a blender. Blend until smooth.

Nutrition Facts Per Serving: Makes 1 serving; Calories 301, Total Fat 7 grams, Saturated Fat 1 gram, Carbohydrates 56 grams, Fiber 11 grams, Protein 10 grams, Sodium 140 milligrams Count as: 2 Flushers/Anti-Bloaters, 1 Protein Slimmer

Zucchini and Tomato Frittata

෴

This frittata is wonderful for breakfast or an elegant brunch. Zucchini and Tomato Frittata combines savory seasonings with fresh garden vegetables for a delightful dish.

1 teaspoon olive oil

1 medium zucchini cut in half lengthwise, then into ¼-inch slices

1 tomato, chopped

2 teaspoons McCormick Onions, Minced

½ teaspoon McCormick Garlic Powder

¼ teaspoon McCormick Thyme Leaves

⅛ teaspoon McCormick Black Pepper, Ground

3 eggs

½ cup shredded cheddar cheese

Heat oil in 9-inch nonstick skillet on medium-high heat. Add zucchini; cook and stir 2 minutes. Add tomato, minced onion, garlic powder, seasoned salt, thyme leaves, and pepper; cook and stir 1 minute.

Beat eggs in medium bowl. Pour over vegetables in skillet. Reduce heat to medium-low; cover and cook 7 minutes.

Sprinkle with cheese. Cover and cook 2 minutes longer or until cheese is melted.

Nutrition Facts Per Serving: Makes 4 servings; Calories 146, Total Fat 10 grams, Carbohydrates 5 grams, Protein 9 grams, Fiber 1 gram, Sodium 77 milligrams
Count as: 1¼ Protein Slimmers, ½ Flusher/Anti-Bloater

From www.mccormick.com

Chicken Salad

⁓

¼ cup celery, chopped

1 tablespoon lemon juice

½ teaspoon onion powder

⅛ teaspoon salt* *(or omit if you prefer)*

3 tablespoons low-fat mayonnaise

3¼ cups skinless chicken breast, cooked, and cubed

Combine all of the ingredients in a large bowl. Mix well and serve.

Nutrition Facts Per Serving: Makes 5 servings; Calories 176, Total Fat 6 grams, Saturated Fat 2 grams, Carbohydrates 2 grams, Protein 27 grams, Fiber 0, Sodium 237 milligrams; *120 milligrams sodium without the added ⅛ teaspoon of salt.
Count as: 1½ Protein Slimmers, 1 Condiment

From The National Heart, Lung, and Blood Institute

Creamy Sun-Dried Tomato Tuna Salad

∽

1 6-ounce can of drained Very Low Sodium or No-Salt-Added Tuna
  (like Starkist Very Low Sodium Tuna)

3 tablespoons nonfat yogurt

2 tablespoons light mayonnaise

5 sprigs basil *(chopped)*

Dash of oregano *(optional)*

10 sundried tomatoes in oil, drained and chopped

2 cups romaine lettuce

Lemon *(optional)*

Mix drained tuna with the yogurt, mayonnaise, basil, and sundried tomatoes. Divide lettuce among two plates and top each with tuna. Spritz with lemon, if desired.

Nutrition Facts Per Serving: Makes 2 servings; Calories 200, Total Fat 11 grams, Saturated Fat 2.5 grams, Carbohydrates 7 grams, Protein 16 grams, Fiber 1 gram, Sodium 230 milligrams Count as: 1½ Protein Slimmers, 1 Flusher/Anti-Bloater, ½ Mono Slimmer

Gold Coast Autumn Salad with California Figs

Lettuce leaves

2 oranges, peeled and thinly sliced

⅔ cup California Dried Figs, Calimyrna or Black Mission, stems removed and quartered

1 apple or ripe pear, cored and thinly sliced

Cardamom Cream Dressing:

½ cup vanilla nonfat yogurt

½ teaspoon honey

¼ teaspoon ground cardamom or cinnamon

1 tablespoon toasted coconut *(garnish)*

On four individual salad plates, arrange a bed of lettuce leaves. Place orange slices, fig quarters, and apple slices decoratively over lettuce. For dressing, in a small bowl, stir together yogurt, honey and ground cardamom until blended. Drizzle mixture over salads. Sprinkle coconut over salads for garnish.

Nutrition Facts Per Serving: Makes 4 servings; Calories 134, Total Fat 1 gram, Saturated Fat 0, Carbohydrates 33 grams, Protein 3 grams, Fiber 5 grams, Sodium 18 grams
Count as: 1¼ Flushers/Anti-Bloaters

From www.californiafigs.com

Harvest Salad with Pork

∾

1 pound pork tenderloin

1 tablespoon I Can't Believe It's Not Butter! spread

1 medium Granny Smith apple, cored and sliced

1 medium onion, sliced

8 cups spring salad mix

½ cup dried cranberries

40 sprays Wish-Bone Salad Spritzers Honey Mustard Dressing

Preheat oven to 425°F. Season pork with black pepper. Place pork in a large roasting pan. Roast 20 minutes or until pork is cooked.

Meanwhile, in 10-inch nonstick skillet, melt I Can't Believe It's Not Butter! spread over medium-high heat and cook apple and onion, stirring frequently, 5 minutes or until golden. Cool slightly.

On serving platter, arrange spring mix. Top with sliced pork, warm apple mixture, and cranberries. Just before serving, spritz with Wish-Bone Salad Spritzers Honey Mustard Dressing

Nutrition Facts Per Serving: Makes 4 servings; Calories 280, Total Fat 10 grams, Saturated Fat 3grams, Carbohydrates 27 grams, Protein 25 grams, Fiber 5 grams, Sodium 203 milligrams Count as: 2 Protein Slimmers, 2 Flushers/Anti-Bloaters

From www.wishbone.com

Shrimp & Corn Salad

∽

Juice of ½ a lemon

1 tablespoon orange juice

¼ cup light mayonnaise

2 teaspoons whole-grain mustard

4 cloves garlic, minced

1 teaspoon canola oil

1 pound shrimp, peeled and deveined

2 cups corn, cut from 2 to 3 cobs

6 cups salad greens

¼ red onion, thinly sliced

1 cup cherry tomatoes, quartered

In a large bowl, whisk together the juices, mayonnaise, and mustard. In a large non-stick skillet over medium heat, sauté the garlic in the oil until golden. Add the shrimp and corn. Sauté until the shrimp are opaque, 2–3 minutes.

Toss the shrimp and corn with the dressing in the bowl. Arrange the salad greens on 4 plates. Top with the shrimp and corn. Garnish with the tomatoes and onion.

Nutrition Facts Per Serving: Makes 4 servings; Calories 270, Total Fat 9 grams, Saturated Fat 1.5 grams, Carbohydrates 22 grams, Protein 26 grams, Fiber 3 grams, Sodium 360 milligrams
Count as: 2 Protein Slimmers, ¾ Carbohydrate Slimmer, 2 Flushers/Anti-Bloaters

From Kate Sherwood

Aromatic Rice

Adding flavor virtually eliminates the need to add salt. This rice is so easy, flavorful, and versatile. It pairs particularly well with your favorite Indian dish.

1 cup basmati brown rice

2 cups water

1 whole cinnamon stick

2 cardamom pods

Combine the rice, water, cinnamon stick, and cardamom pods in a 2-quart saucepan. Bring the mixture to a boil, reduce the heat to a simmer, cover and cook for 20 minutes or until the rice is tender.

Remove the pan from the heat. Fluff with a fork, cover, and let it stand for 10 more minutes.

Nutrition Facts Per ½-Cup Serving: Makes approximately 4 servings; Calories 98, Total Fat 1 gram, Saturated Fat 0, Carbohydrates 21 grams, Protein 2 grams, Fiber 1.5 grams, Sodium 0 Count as: 1 Carbohydrate Slimmer

From Elizabeth Gordon, owner of Betsy & Claude Baking Co., specializing in gluten-free, dairy-, soy-, nut-, and egg-free baked goods. www.betsyandclaude.com

Extra Spicy Potatoes

～

1 large baking potato

1 small onion

Cooking spray

1 teaspoon Mrs. Dash Extra Spicy Seasoning Blend

Dice baking potato and onion. Add potato and onion to medium skillet sprayed with cooking spray. Sprinkle with Mrs. Dash Extra Spicy Seasoning Blend. Sauté until tender.

Nutrition Facts Per Serving: Makes 2 servings; Calories 152, Total Fat 0, Saturated Fat 0, Carbohydrates 35 grams, Protein 4 grams, Fiber 4 grams, Sodium 16 milligrams
Count as: 1½ Carbohydrate Slimmers

From www.MrsDash.com

Mushroom Barley Risotto

⌒⌒

4 cups fat-free low-sodium chicken or vegetable broth
2 tablespoons olive oil
1 small onion, chopped
3 cups pearl barley, sorted and rinsed
1 cup dry white wine
1 pound Portabella or white button mushrooms, trimmed and sliced
2 tablespoons chopped shallots
2 tablespoons chopped fresh basil
3 tablespoons grated Parmesan cheese
Salt *(optional, use cautiously)*

In a saucepan, bring the broth to a boil. Cover the pan and turn off the heat.

Heat 1 tablespoon of the olive oil in a deep skillet over medium heat. Add the onion and sauté until soft. Reduce the heat to low. Add the barley and stir it to coat with oil. Add the wine and cook, stirring, until wine is absorbed. Add the hot broth, ½ cup at a time, stirring frequently and adding ½ cup more of broth each time the previous addition is almost absorbed. This should take about 30 minutes. (You may have a little broth left over.) If the barley is not yet tender and all the broth is gone, add a little water and cook until it is tender.

Put remaining 1 tablespoon of the olive oil in a skillet over a medium-high flame. Add the mushrooms and shallots, and sauté until mushrooms are golden and shallots are soft, about 5 minutes. (If the mixture begins to stick, remove the skillet from the flame and spray the mushrooms with nonstick cooking spray. Return the skillet to the heat and cook until the mushrooms are golden and shallots are soft.)

Stir the mushroom mixture and basil into the barley. Season with salt and pepper. Serve immediately, with a sprinkle of Parmesan cheese.

Nutrition Facts Per Serving: Makes 4 servings; Calories 257, Total Fat 8 grams, Saturated Fat 2 grams, Carbohydrates 36 grams, Protein 8 grams, Fiber 2 grams, Sodium 167 milligrams
Count as: 2 Carbohydrate Slimmers, 1 Mono Slimmer, 1 Flusher/Anti-Bloater

From www.mushroominfo.com and http://www.themushroomchannel.com/

The Nutrition Twins Skinny Cauliflower Mash

⌒∕◌

1 head cauliflower
⅛ cup skim milk
2 cloves garlic, chopped
Pepper, to taste
Butter spray *(10 sprays)*

Steam cauliflower until tender when poked with a fork. Place cauliflower (pieces), skim milk, garlic, and pepper in a blender. Blend until smooth. Place mixture in a small baking dish and sprinkle with paprika, if desired. Bake at 350 degrees in oven until bubbly.

Nutrition Facts Per Serving: Makes 3 servings; Calories 32.6, Total Fat 1 gram, Saturated Fat 0.1 gram, Carbohydrates 5.7 grams, Protein 2.7 grams, Fiber 0, Sodium 34.2 milligrams
Count as: 2 Flushers/Anti-Bloaters

The Nutrition Twins Skinny Mashed Potatoes

ை

2 small red-skin potatoes *(together, they should be smaller than the size of your fist [1-inch diameter each, approximately 3 ounces total])*

2 tablespoons The Nutrition Twins Skinny Anti-Bloat Broth or Campbell's Low-Sodium Chicken Broth

I Can't Believe It's Not Butter! spray *(optional)*

1 teaspoon grated Parmesan

Bring a saucepan of water to a boil. Add potatoes, leaving skin intact, and cook until tender but still firm (about 10 minutes). Drain, and place in a large bowl.

Combine potatoes with chicken broth. Mash together until smooth and creamy. Spray It's Not Butter! spray, and sprinkle grated Parmesan, if desired.

For a salternative: After transferring the cooked, tender potatoes to a large bowl, immediately add a chopped clove of garlic (or garlic powder), a sprinkle of dried oregano and a teaspoon of grated Romano cheese.

Nutrition Facts Per Serving: Makes 1 serving; Calories 120, Total Fat 1 gram, Saturated Fat 0, Carbohydrates 27 grams, Protein 4 grams, Fiber 2.5 grams, Sodium 35 grams
Count as: 1 Carbohydrate Slimmers

The Nutrition Twins Skinny Rice Pilaf

∽

1 cup brown rice

1 cup green onion, chopped finely

1½ cups fat-free, low-sodium vegetable or chicken broth

¼ cup toasted almonds, chopped finely

Add all ingredients except for almonds into a rice cooker and press Start. When the rice is finished, stir in almonds.

Nutrition Facts Per Serving: Makes 4 servings; Calories 150, Total Fat 3 grams, Saturated Fat 0, Carbohydrates 25 grams, Protein 5 grams, Fiber 3 grams, Sodium 20 milligrams
Count as: 1½ Carbohydrate Slimmers

The Nutrition Twins Skinny Spinach You Can Sink Your Teeth Into

❧

1 10-ounce package frozen spinach or 1 bag raw spinach
  (9- to 10-ounce bag)
¾ cup Walnut Acres low-sodium Tomato and Basil Pasta sauce
  (or other low-sodium tomato sauce with less than 40 calories per serving)
1 tablespoon nonfat mozzarella cheese
2 teaspoons grated Parmesan cheese

Steam fresh spinach or prepare frozen spinach according to directions on package. Heat tomato sauce and then stir into spinach. Add cheese and stir. Divide spinach into two portions and sprinkle with Parmesan.

Nutrition Facts Per Serving: Makes 2 servings; Calories 86, Total Fat 2 grams, Saturated Fat 1 gram, Carbohydrates 14 grams, Protein 5.5 grams, Fiber 5 grams, Sodium 169 milligrams
Count as: 2½ Flushers/Anti-Bloaters, ¼ Protein Slimmer

The Nutrition Twins Skinny Anti-Bloat Broth

∽

After preparing the broth, pour it into ice cube trays and store the trays in the freezer. Anytime you sauté anything, from veggies to meats, pop out a cube and your low-sodium broth is conveniently ready. Note: When preparing the broth, keep the lid on the pot the entire time so the nutrients remain in the water and don't boil out.

5 cloves of garlic, pressed

1 large carrot *(scrubbed and cut into ½-inch slices)*

1 stalk of bok choy *(cut into ½-inch slices) (optional)*

2 large celery stalks *(cut into ½-inch slices)*

1 medium yellow onion *(cut into large pieces)*

2 large bay leaves

10 sprigs fresh parsley *(left whole)*

1 mushroom, sliced

8 cups water

Place all ingredients in a large pot filled with cold water. Put a lid on the pot and bring to a boil. When broth boils, lower the heat to low and continue cooking, covered, for 45 minutes to 1 hour.

Once it's cooled, strain the broth. Store the broth in an airtight container in either the refrigerator (where it will keep for several days) or freezer (where it will stay good for several months). Discard the cooked vegetables and other remaining ingredients.

Nutrition Facts Per Serving: Makes 8 1-cup servings; Calories 18, Total Fat 0 gram, Saturated Fat 0, Carbohydrates 4 grams, Protein 1 gram, Fiber 1 gram, Sodium 19 milligrams
Count as: 1 Freebie

Thai Pumpkin Soup

∾

Fresh ginger and creamy peanut butter lend a distinct Thai flavor to this soup. Serve with a mixed green salad and mango slices drizzled with honey.

2 cups water

1 15-ounce can 100% Pure Pumpkin

1 11.5-ounce can mango nectar

3 Vegetable Flavor Bouillon Cubes

1 teaspoon finely chopped fresh ginger or ¾ teaspoon ground ginger

2½ cloves garlic, finely chopped

½ teaspoon crushed red pepper

¼ cup creamy peanut butter

2 tablespoons rice vinegar

3 tablespoons finely chopped green onion

⅔ cup *(5-ounce can)* Evaporated Fat Free Milk

Combine water, pumpkin, nectar, bouillon, ginger, garlic and crushed red pepper in large saucepan. Bring to a boil, stirring occasionally. Reduce heat to low.

Stir in peanut butter, vinegar, and green onion. Cook, stirring occasionally, for 5 to 8 minutes or until soup returns to a boil. Stir in evaporated milk.

FOR FREEZE AHEAD: Prepare as above. Cool soup completely. Place in airtight container; freeze for up to 2 months. Thaw overnight in refrigerator.

Heat in medium saucepan over medium heat, stirring occasionally, for 15 to 20 minutes or until heated through.

Nutrition Facts Per Serving: Makes 4 servings; Calories 220, Total Fat 9 grams, Saturated Fat 1.5 grams, Carbohydrates 31 grams, Protein 9 grams, Fiber 6 grams, Sodium 160 milligrams
Count as: 1 Carbohydrate Slimmer, 1 Protein Slimmer, ⅓ Mono Slimmer

Vegetarian Spaghetti Sauce

2 tablespoons olive oil

2 small onions, chopped

3 cloves garlic, chopped

1¼ cups zucchini, sliced

1 tablespoon oregano, dried

1 tablespoon basil, dried

1 8-ounce can tomato sauce

1 6-ounce can low-sodium tomato paste

2 medium tomatoes, chopped

1 cup water

In a medium skillet, heat oil. Sauté onions, garlic, and zucchini in oil for 5 minutes on medium heat.

Add remaining ingredients and simmer covered for 45 minutes. Serve over spaghetti.

Nutrition Facts Per Serving: Makes 6 servings; Calories 105, Total Fat 5 grams, Saturated Fat 1 gram, Carbohydrates 15 grams, Protein 3 grams, Fiber 4 grams, Sodium 253 milligrams
Count as: 1 Carbohydrate Slimmer

From The National Heart, Lung, and Blood Institute

Vinaigrette Salad Dressing

1 bulb garlic, separated and peeled

½ cup water

1 tablespoon red wine vinegar

¼ teaspoon honey

1 tablespoon virgin olive oil

¼ teaspoon black pepper

Place the garlic cloves into a small saucepan and pour in enough water (about ½ cup) to cover them. Bring water to a boil, then reduce heat and simmer until garlic is tender, about 15 minutes.

Reduce the liquid to 2 tablespoons and increase the heat for 3 minutes. Pour the contents into a small sieve over a bowl, and with a wooden spoon, mash the garlic through the sieve into the bowl. Whisk the vinegar and honey into the garlic mixture; incorporate the oil and seasoning.

Nutrition Facts Per Serving: (2 tablespoons): Makes 4 servings; Calories 33, Total Fat 3 grams, Saturated Fat 0 gram, Carbohydrate 1 gram, Protein 0, Fiber 0, Sodium 1 milligram
Count as: 3 Freebies or 1 Condiment

From The National Heart, Lung, and Blood Institute

Applesauce Oatmeal Cookies

∽

1 cup whole wheat flour

3 cup oatmeal (instant, cooked)

1 teaspoon baking soda

¼ teaspoon nutmeg

1 cup unsweetened applesauce

1 cup sugar (or less)

1 teaspoon vanilla

⅔ cup raisins or dried apples

Combine the flour, oatmeal, baking soda and nutmeg. Then mix the applesauce, sugar, and vanilla together and add them to the oatmeal mixture. Stir in the dried fruit. Roll in small balls and smash to ¼ inch thickness on the cookie sheet. Bake at 275°F for 22–25 minutes.

Nutrition Facts per Serving (per cookie): Makes about 25 cookies; Calories 88, Total Fat .5 grams, Saturated Fat 0 grams, Carbohydrate 20 grams, Protein 1.5 grams, Fiber 2 grams, Sodium 70 milligrams
Count as: 1 Red Light Food

Blueberry Almond Biscotti

Blueberries have long been known to have powerful antioxidant qualities, and research has shown that eating fruits naturally high in antioxidants helps to slow age-related health problems. Pair dried blueberries with heart-healthy raw almonds for a heart-healthy treat.

2 eggs

⅔ cup sugar

1 teaspoon almond extract

¾ cups flour

½ teaspoon baking soda

¼ teaspoon salt

1 *(3½-ounce)* bag Sunsweet Dried Blueberries

½ cup shredded or flake coconut

½ cup whole raw almonds

Preheat oven to 350°F and line a baking sheet with parchment paper. Beat eggs, sugar, and extract together in a medium bowl. Add flour, baking soda, and salt, stirring to form a stiff dough. Stir in blueberries, coconut, and almonds.

Shape dough into a ball on a floured board. Press into a 10 x 7-inch rectangle (about ½-inch thick) on prepared baking sheet. Bake for 30 minutes; let cool slightly.

Cut into very thin slices with a serrated knife, and place on 2 baking sheets. Reduce heat to 200°F and bake for 12 to 15 minutes on each side or until just starting to brown around the edges. Let cool completely to crisp.

Nutrition Facts Per Serving (1 biscotti): Makes about 40 servings; Calories 120, Fat 3.5 grams, Saturated Fat 1 gram, Carbohydrates 21 grams, Protein 3 grams, Fiber 2 grams, Sodium 75 milligrams Count as: ¼ Flusher/Anti-Bloater, ¼ Mono-Slimmer, ½ Red Light Food

From Sunsweet Growers, Inc.

Fudgy Brownies

½ cup unbleached all-purpose flour

¾ cup unsweetened cocoa powder

½ teaspoon baking powder

¼ teaspoon salt

3 egg whites

2 whole eggs

1 cup granulated sugar

½ cup brown sugar

⅔ cup unsweetened applesauce

2 teaspoons vanilla extract

¼ cup crushed nuts (any nut of your choice)

Preheat oven to 350°F (180°C). Grease a 13" x 9" (32.5 x 23-cm) baking pan.

Combine the flour, cocoa powder, baking powder, and salt in a medium-size bowl.

In a large bowl, beat the egg whites with an electric beater until foamy. Gently stir in the eggs, granulated sugar, and brown sugar until well-combined. Blend in the applesauce and vanilla extract. Stir in the flour mixture.

Spread the batter into the pan and sprinkle with nuts. Bake for about 30 minutes or until a fork inserted in the middle comes out clean. Do not over bake. Cool the brownies in the pan on a rack.

Nutrition facts per serving (one brownie): Makes 32 brownies; Calories 71, Total Fat 2 grams, Carbohydrates 13 grams, Protein 2 grams, Fiber 1 gram, Sodium 37 milligrams
Count as: ¾ Red Light Food

Appendix I:
The Jumpstart Plan Food Lists
(Brand-Name Green Light Foods)

List A: Carbohydrate Slimmers
(Count Each as 1 Carb Slimmer Unless Noted)

Food	Serving Size	Calories	Fiber (gm)	Sodium (mg)
BREADS				
Alvarado Street Bakery No Salt! Sprouted Multi-grain Bread	1 slice (34 grams)	90	2	10
Cinnamon Raisin Gnu Bar[1], [1.5 Carbohydrate Slimmers]	1 bar	130	12	30
Ezekiel 4:9 Organic Sprouted Whole Grain Sesame Bread	1 slice (34 grams)	80	3	80
Natural Ovens Bakery Whole Grain Naturals	1 slice (36 grams)	100	4	110
Pepperidge Farm Stoneground 100% Whole Wheat	1 small slice or (1 oz)	70	2	100
Pepperidge Farm Whole Grain 100% Whole Wheat small	1 small slice or (1 oz)	70	2	100

[1]*Gnu bars are actually bars, not bread, but they're made from whole grains. Unlike most bars, they're so wholesome, fiber-packed and low in sodium (only 30–42 mg sodium and 130 calories in Cinnamon Raisin, Orange Cranberry and Banana; 140 calories for the Peanut Butter Bar and the Chocolate Brownie Bar) that they qualify as 1.5 Carbohydrate Slimmers. Plus, they don't have high fructose corn syrup added like many breads.*

Carb Slimmers Continued *(Count Each as 1 Carb Slimmer Unless Noted)*

Food	Serving Size	Calories	Fiber (gm)	Sodium (mg)
LIGHT OR LOW-CALORIE BREADS 1-Slice = (About ¾ oz)				
Arnold or Brownberry Bakery Light 100% Whole Wheat	1 slice (¾ oz)	40	3	100
Natural Ovens Bakery Weight Sense Right Wheat	1 slice (¾ oz)	50	3	70
Nature's Own 100% Whole Grain Wheat Sugar Free	1 slice (¾ oz)	50	2	110
Sara Lee 45 Calories and Delightful—100% Multi-Grain or 100% Whole Wheat with Honey	1 slice (¾ oz)	50	2	110
Weight Watchers 100% Whole Wheat	1 slice (¾ oz)	50	3	90
PITA				
Trader Joe's 100% Whole Wheat Apocryphal Pita [1.5 Slimmers]	2 oz	140	4	110
Trader Joe's Organic 100% Whole Wheat Pita	1 oz	80	2	60
TORTILLAS/WRAPS				
Corn Tortillas	2 tortillas (38 gm)	82	3	17
Lavash All Natural Roll Ups	1 wrap (1.5 oz)	110	4	30
Tumaro's Gourmet Tortillas-Soy-ful Heart Flatbread	1 tortilla (1.4 oz)	90	4	65

Carb Slimmers Continued *(Count Each as 1 Carb Slimmer Unless Noted)*

Food	Serving Size	Calories	Fiber (gm)	Sodium (mg)
RICE AND PASTA				
Brown Rice	½ cup cooked	108	2	2
Whole Wheat Pasta	½ cup cooked	87	2	0
CRACKERS				
Health Valley Rice Bran Graham Crackers, Original	6 crackers (28 gm)	110	3	70
Matzo, Whole Wheat	1 slice (28 gm)	98	3	1
CRISPBREAD				
GG Bran Scandinavian Crispbread	1 slice (10 gm)	12	5	30
Ryvita Dark Rye Crispbread	1 slice (10 gm)	35	2	40
Ryvita Fruit Crunch Crispbread	2 slices	100	4	0
Ryvita Light Rye Crispbread	1 slice (10 gm)	35	2	20
Ryvita Multigrain Crispbread	1 slice (11 gm)	45	2	45
Ryvita Rye and Oat Bran Crispbread	1 slice (10 gm)	35	2	10
Ryvita Sesame Rye Crispbread	1 slice (10 gm)	40	2	40
POPCORN				
Popcorn, air-popped (no oil, no butter added)	3 cups popped	93	3.5	2
Jolly Time Low Sodium 100 Calorie Healthy Pop Butter	1 bag	100	8	90
Smart Balance Smart 'n Healthy Microwave Popcorn	5 cups popped	120	5	85

Carb Slimmers Continued *(Count Each as 1 Carb Slimmer Unless Noted)*

Food	Serving Size	Calories	Fiber (gm)	Sodium (mg)
BEANS AND LEGUMES				
Edamame (Soybeans) fresh, boiled, drained with pods, no salt added [Count as either a Carb Slimmer or a Protein Slimmer]	½ cup	75	5	4
Edamame (Soybeans) fresh, boiled, drained, without pods, no salt added [Count as either a Carb Slimmer or a Protein Slimmer]	⅓ cup	85	2.5	8
Legumes, lentils, and split peas; (not green beans) canned "no salt" or "low sodium" canned, rinsed [Count as either a Carb Slimmer or a Protein Slimmer]	½ cup canned	100	5.5	10
Legumes, lentils, and split peas) (not green beans); dried, no salt added [Count as either a Carb Slimmer or a Protein Slimmer]	⅔ cup	80	3.7	3
STARCHY VEGGIES				
Corn; fresh or frozen, boiled and drained, no salt added) (Starchy Veggie)	1 ear fresh or ¾ cup	100	3	17
Peas; fresh, boiled, and drained (no salt added) (Starchy Veggie)	¾ cup	95	6.6	3 (80 mg for frozen)
Potato, sweet or white fresh, cooked, with skin, no salt added (Starchy Veggie)	½ cup or 3.5 oz	90	3.3	32

Carb Slimmers Continued *(Count Each as 1 Carb Slimmer Unless Noted)*

Food	Serving Size	Calories	Fiber (gm)	Sodium (mg)
STARCHY VEGGIES *continued*				
Ore-Ida Steam n' Mash Cut Sweet Potatoes (Starchy Veggie)	1 cup of mini potato chunks	90	3	30
Squash, acorn (Starchy Veggie)	1 cup	112	8	8
Squash, butternut, fresh, baked, no salt (1 cup) (Starchy Veggie)	1 cup	100	3	8
TOMATO SAUCE				
Eden No Salt Added Spaghetti Sauce (Starchy Veggie)	½ cup	80	3	10
Enricos All Natural No Salt Added Pasta Sauce (Starchy Veggie)	½ cup	60	1	25
Manischewitz No Salt Added Marinara Pasta Sauce (Starchy Veggie)	½ cup	70	2	45
Rokeach No Salt Added Tomato Sauce with Mushrooms (Starchy Veggie)	½ cup	80	3	50

Carb Slimmers Continued *(Count Each as 1 Carb Slimmer Unless Noted)*

Food	Serving Size	Calories	Fiber (gm)	Sodium (mg)	Sugar (mg)
CEREAL					
All Bran	31 gm	80	10	80	6
Fiber One	30 gm	60	14	105	0
Go Lean [1.5 Slimmers]	52 gm	140	10	85	6
Go Lean [2 Slimmers]	53 gm	190	8	95	13
Kashi 7 Whole Grain Flakes [2 Slimmers]	50 gm	180	6	150	5
Kashi Heart to Heart	33 gm	110	5	90	5
Kashi Vive, Toasted Graham & Vanilla [2 Slimmers]	55 gm	170	12	100	10
Nature's Path Organic Synergy 8 Whole Grains	¾ cup (30 gm)	100	5	0	4
Post Shredded Wheat Spoon Size [2 Slimmers]	49 gm	170	6	0	0
HOT CEREALS					
Country Choice Organic Original Plain Instant Oatmeal	1 packet (29 gm)	110	3	0	1
Kashi Instant Oatmeal, Apple Cinnamon [2 Slimmers]	1 packet (43 gm)	160	5	110	12
Kashi Instant Oatmeal, Golden Brown Maple [2 Slimmers]	1 packet (43 gm)	160	5	100	12
Quaker Instant Oatmeal, Regular	1 packet (28 gm)	100	3	80	0

Carb Slimmers Continued *(Count Each as 1 Carb Slimmer Unless Noted)*

Food	Serving Size	Calories	Fiber (gm)	Sodium (mg)	Sugar (mg)
HOT CEREALS *continued*					
Quaker Instant Organic Regular	1 packet (28 gm)	100	3	0	0
Quaker Old Fashioned Oats [1.5 Slimmers]	½ cup (dry) (40 gm)	150	4	0	1
Quaker Instant Oatmeal, Take Heart, Golden Maple [2 Slimmers]	1 packet (45 gm)	160	5	110	9
Quaker Instant Oatmeal, Apple Cinnamon [1.5 Slimmers]	1 packet (35 gm)	130	3	170	12
Quaker Oat Bran Hot Cereal [1.5 Slimmers]	1 packet (35 gm)	150	6	0	1
Zoe's Cinnamon Raisin Granola [2 Slimmers]	¾ cup (50 gm)	190	7	70	12

List B: Protein Slimmers
(Count as 1 Protein Slimmer Unless Noted)

Food	Serving Size	Calories	Sodium (mg)
BEANS			
Legumes, Lentils, and Split Peas, (not green beans), canned "low sodium" or "no salt added"	½ cup	100	10
Legumes, Lentils, and Split Peas, (not green beans), dried, "low sodium" or "no salt added"	⅔ cup	80	3

Protein Slimmers Continued *(Count Each as 1 Protein Slimmer Unless Noted)*

Food	Serving Size	Calories	Sodium (mg)
BEANS *continued*			
Eden Cajun Small Red Beans And Rice	½ cup	110	115
Eden Caribbean Black Beans And Rice	½ cup	120	100
Eden Organic Black Beans	½ cup	110	15
Eden Organic Black Eyed Peas	½ cup	90	25
Eden Organic Kidney Beans	½ cup	100	15
SOY ITEMS			
Soybeans (Edamame) no salt added, without pods	30 pods or ⅓ cup without pods	85	8
Tempeh, Not Fried	½ cup	110	7
Tofu, Not Fried	½ cup	100	8
MEAT			
Red Meats, Extra Lean Only, Fresh, Cooked, Not Fried) (red meat: the round and the loin; pork: the tenderloin, all fat removed)	1.5 ounces	95	19
Poultry Breasts, Skinless, Fresh, Cooked (not fried)	2 ounces	94	32
Boneless, Skinless Chicken Breast Cooked Tenderloins	2 ounces	68	17
Poultry Breast, Deli Sliced ("low-sodium" only)	2 ounces	60–80	≤350
Boar's Head 47% Less Sodium	2 ounces	60	340
HARVESTLAND Boneless, Skinless Chicken Breasts	2 ounces	55	30
Jennie-O Low-Sodium Turkey Breast	2 ounces	50	260

Several meats on the Protein Slimmers list are higher in calories despite being Slimmers. These meats are starred on List B. Use the specific serving sizes listed for them.

Protein Slimmers Continued *(Count Each as 1 Protein Slimmer Unless Noted)*

Food	Serving Size	Calories	Sodium (mg)
MEATS *continued*			
Perdue Fit & Easy Fresh Ground Chicken Breast, cooked	2 ounces	52	41
Perdue, Fit & Easy Boneless, Skinless Chicken Cooked Breast	2 ounces	55	23
Sara Lee Lower Sodium Oven Roasted Turkey Breast	2 ounces	50	340
FISH			
Fish, Fresh, no skin, cooked, dry heat, not fried (except salmon, anchovies and sardines)	2 ounces	55–90	30–70
Fish, Canned, in water only, low sodium, no salt added, and very low sodium only	2 ounces	60–120	15–100
Salmon, fresh, no skin, fresh cooked, not fried	1.5 ounces	95	28
Oysters, cooked, moist heat, no added salt or sauce	2 ounces	45	93
Squid (calamari), steamed, not fried; no salt, no sauce	2 ounces	65	31
Shellfish (Shrimp, Clams, Scallops), [Not Alaskan King Crab, Lobster, Mussels], fresh, cooked dry heat, not fried (Limit shellfish to twice a week)	2 ounces	55 (shrimp); 62 (scallops); 83 (clams)	115 (shrimp); 130 (scallops); 62 (clams)
MILK			
Milk, Skim and 1% only	1 cup	90 (skim); 105 (1%) calories	130
Soy milk	1 cup	70–100	80–140

Protein Slimmers Continued *(Count Each as 1 Protein Slimmer Unless Noted)*

Food	Serving Size	Calories	Sodium (mg)
EGGS			
Egg Beaters	½ cup	60	230
Egg whites	4 whites	70	200
Hard-boiled	4 whites	75	62
COTTAGE CHEESE, LOW-FAT AND NONFAT ONLY Sodium (380 mg or less)			
Cottage Cheese, nonfat or low-fat, limit to one serving a day (like Friendship brand)	½ cup	80	≤380
Cottage Cheese, nonfat or low-fat, low sodium (like Friendship brand)	½ cup	90	50
Ricotta Cheese, Fat Free, Frigo	½ cup	80	300

Food	Serving Size	Calories	Sodium (≤240 mg)	Fat (≤3 grams)
COTTAGE CHEESE, LOW FAT AND NONFAT ONLY				
Cabot, Cheddar, 75% Light	1 ounce	60	200	2.5
Farmer's Cheese (average of most brands)	1 ounce	50	120	2.5
Lifetime, Low-Fat Cheddar Slices	1 slice	30	180	1
Polly-O Fat Free Mozzarella Cheese	1 ounce	35	220	0
Sargento Light String Cheese	.7 ounce	50	180	2.5
Smart Beat, Cheese Substitute, Cheddar, Fat Free	1 slice	25	180	0

Be cautious: cheese varies from 90–500 mg per ounce. Only choose cheeses with 240 mgr or less of sodiuun per ounce.

Protein Slimmers Continued *(Count Each as 1 Protein Slimmer Unless Noted)*

Food	Serving Size	Calories	Sodium (≤240 mg)	Fat (≤3 grams)
COTTAGE CHEESE, LOW FAT AND NONFAT ONLY *continued*				
Swiss Cheese, Low-Fat (average of most brands)	1 ounce	50	73	1.5
The Laughing Cow, Mini Babybel, Light Original (Avoid other flavors—they have 100 mg more sodium)	1 piece	50	160	3
Trader Joe Light Organic String Cheese	1 ounce	60	180	2.5
Wegman's Low-Fat Goat Cheese	1 ounce	45	100	3

Be cautious: cheese varies from 90–500 mg per ounce. Only choose cheeses with 240 mg or less of sodiuun per ounce.

Food	Serving Size	Calories	Sodium (≤240 mg)	Fat (≤3 grams)
SOY CHEESE				
Galaxy Veggie Slices, American Flavor	1 slice	30	220	2.5
Smart Beat: Soy Smart Slices American Cheese	1 slice	25	180	0
Soy Sation Soy Cheese Shredded Mozzarella and Cheddar	1 slice	63	190	3
Trader Joe's Soy Cheese, Cheddar Flavor only	1 slice	45	180	2

Protein Slimmers Continued *(Count Each as 1 Protein Slimmer Unless Noted)*

Food	Calories (≤100 cal)	Total Fat (≤3 gm)	Sugars (≤12 gm)	Protein (≤5 gm)	Calcium (≤10% DV)
YOGURT					
Nonfat Plain, any brand, (6 oz)	80	0	12	8	30
Dannon Light and Fit (6 oz) (Note: Strawberry only has 15% calcium DV)	80	0	11	5	20
0% Fage Greek Style Yogurt (5.3 oz)	80	0	6	13	10
Oikos Organic Greek Style Yogurt (5.3 oz)	80	0	6	15	20

List C: Mono Slimmers
(Each Item Listed Below Equals 1 Mono Slimmer)

Mono Slimmers	Serving Size	Calories	Sodium
OILS: Olive, Flaxseed, Peanut, Walnut, Sunflower, Sesame	3 teaspoons	120	0
NUTS AND SEEDS, UNSALTED			
Almonds	14 nuts	100	0
Almond Butter	3 level teaspoons	100	0
Brazil Nuts	4 nuts	100	1
Cashews, dry or oil roasted	11 nuts	99	3
Chestnuts	¼ cup	100	0
Filberts/Hazelnuts	11 nuts	100	0
Flaxseeds	2 tablespoons	100	10
Macadamias	5 nuts or ½ tbsp	102	2
Mixed Nuts	2 tablespoons	100	2

Protein Slimmers Continued *(Count Each as 1 Protein Slimmer Unless Noted)*

Mono Slimmers	Serving Size	Calories	Sodium
Peanut butter (unsalted)	1 level tbsp	100	0
Peanuts	20 nuts	100	0
Pecans, dry or oil roasted	7 halves	100	1
Pine Nuts, dried	6 teaspoons	100	1
Pistachios	30 nuts	100	0
Pumpkin Kernels, dried	2 tablespoons	100	1
Sesame Seeds	2 tablespoons	100	0
Sunflower Seeds, dry or oil roasted	2 tablespoons	93	0
NUT BUTTERS (unsalted) and TAHINI	3 level teaspoons	100	0
Avocado, pureed	¼ cup or 4 level tablespoons or ¼ small avocado	100	0
Hummus	3 level tablespoons	100	Choose brands with 150 mg or less for 3 tblsp

List D: Flushers and Anti-Bloaters

All vegetables and fruits qualify as Flushers and Anti-Bloaters; however, the most potent ones are labeled as Flushers or Anti-Bloaters. Those fruits and vegetables that aren't labeled are still great Flushers and Anti-Bloaters, just not the most powerful ones. Here are some examples:

Vegetables		
Asparagus (Anti-Bloater)	Brussels sprouts (Flusher)	Celery
Artichokes (Anti-Bloater)	Bok choy (Anti-Bloater)	Collard greens (Anti-Bloater)
Beets (Anti-Bloater)	Cabbage (Flusher)	Cucumbers (Anti-Bloater)
Bell peppers (Flusher)	Carrots (Flusher)	Eggplant
Broccoli (Flusher)	Cauliflower (Flusher)	Fennel

Green beans

Green peas

Greens: beet, collard, mustard, turnip (Anti-Bloater)

Kale (Anti-Bloater)

Leeks

Mushrooms

Mustard greens (Flusher, Anti-Bloater)

Onions

Parsley (Anti-Bloater)

Pumpkin (Flusher)

Romaine lettuce

Spinach (Flusher, Anti-Bloater)

Squash, spaghetti (Flusher)

Squash, yellow

String beans

Swiss chard

Tomatoes (Anti-Bloater, See list of tomato sauces on page XX that qualify as Anti-Bloaters)

Turnip greens (Flusher, Anti-Bloater)

Zucchini

Fruits

Apples (Flusher)

Apricots (Anti-Bloater)

Bananas (Anti-Bloater)

Blackberries (Flusher)

Blueberries (Flusher)

Boysenberries (Flusher)

Cantaloupe (Anti-Bloater)

Cranberries (Anti-Bloater)

Currants (Flusher)

Elderberries (Flusher)

Figs (Flusher)

Gooseberries

Grapefruit (Anti-Bloater)

Grapes

Honeydew (Anti-Bloater)

Kiwifruit (Flusher, Anti-Bloater)

Lemon/Limes (Anti-Bloater)

Logan Berries (Flusher)

Mango (Anti-Bloater)

Nectarines (Anti-Bloater)

Oranges (Flusher, Anti-Bloater)

Papaya (Anti-Bloater)

Pears (Flusher, Anti-Bloater)

Peaches (Anti-Bloater)

Pineapple

Plums (Anti-Bloater)

Plums, dried (prunes) (Flusher)

Raisins (Flusher, Anti-Bloater)

Raspberries (Flusher)

Strawberries (Flusher)

Watermelon (Anti-Bloater)

The following non-starchy tomato sauces are Anti-Bloaters.

Food	Serving Size	Calories	Sodium (mg)	Fiber (gm)
Del Monte Tomato Sauce No Salt Added	½ cup	40	40	1
Roselli's No Added Sugar Low Sodium Spaghetti Sauce	½ cup	35	45	2
Walnut Acres Low Sodium Tomato and Basil Pasta Sauce	½ cup	40	20	1

Appendix II: The Maintenance Plan Food Lists (Brand-Name Green Light and Yellow Light Foods)

List A (Phase II): What Additional Carbohydrate Slimmers Can I Eat Now?

Food	Calories	Fiber (gm)	Sodium (mg)
BREADS (Most are 1.5 oz unless noted)			
Arnold Light Whole Wheat Bread (2 slices = 1 serving) [1 Slimmer]	80	5	150
Arnold or Brownberry Bakery 100% Whole Wheat [1 Slimmer]	70	2	140
Freihofer's, Whole Wheat (1 slice, 36 gm) [1 Slimmer]	90	2	160
Home Pride Whole Grains Honey Whole Wheat (1 oz) [1 Slimmer]	80	2	150
Natural Ovens 100% Whole Wheat Bread [1 Slimmer]	120	4	130
Natural Ovens Bakery Organic PLUS 100% Whole Wheat [1 Slimmer]	120	4	130
Pepperidge Farm Farmhouse Soft 100% Whole Wheat [1 Slimmer]	110	3	150
*Pepperidge Farm Very Thin Soft 100% Whole Wheat (2 slices) [1 Slimmer]	80	2	160

* The bread is listed as two slices; one slice wouldn't have enough fiber. Plus, in most instances, one slice won't fill you and you'd most likely be hungry, making it difficult to stay on track.

Food	Calories	Fiber (gm)	Sodium (mg)
BREADS (Most are 1.5 oz unless noted)			
Pepperidge Farm Whole Grain 100% Whole Wheat [1 Slimmer]	110	3	150
Pepperidge Farm Whole Grain 15 Grain Small Slice (1 oz) [1 Slimmer]	80	2	120
Pepperidge Farm Whole Grain Oatmeal Small Slice (1 oz) [1 Slimmer]	70	2	120
Pepperidge Farm Whole Grain Swirl [1 Slimmer]	100	3	150
Sara Lee Heart Healthy Classic 100% Whole Wheat [1 Slimmer]	70	2	130
Sara Lee Soft & Smooth 100% Honey Wheat (1 oz) [1 Slimmer]	70	2	130
Sara Lee Soft & Smooth 100% Whole Wheat (1 oz) [1 Slimmer]	70	2	140
Stroehmann Dutch Country 100% Whole Wheat, Stone Ground (1 slice, 38 gm) [1 Slimmer]	100	3	200
Weight Watchers, Whole Wheat (2 slices = 1 serving) [1 Slimmer]	90	5	180
Wonder 100% Whole Grain (1 oz) [1 Slimmer]	80	2	150
PITA			
Thomas' Sahara Pita Pockets 100% Whole Wheat or Multi-grain (1 2-oz Pita Pocket) [1 Yellow Light Food, 0.5 Slimmer]	140	4	320
Toufayan Whole Wheat Pita (2 oz) [1.5 Slimmers]	140	3	130
Trader Joe's 100% Whole Wheat Apocryphal Pita (2 oz) [1.5 Slimmers]	140	4	110
Weight Watchers 100% Whole Wheat Pita (2 oz) [1 Yellow Light Food]	100	9	260

Food	Calories	Fiber (gm)	Sodium (mg)
TORTILLAS/WRAPS			
Flatout Wraps Mini-Harvest Whole Wheat or 100% Stone Ground Whole Wheat (1 oz) [1 Slimmer]	70	3	190
Flatout Wraps Whole Grain White (2 oz) [1 Yellow Light Food]	110	7	350
La Tortilla Factory Whole Wheat Grain Wrap [1 Yellow Light Food]	120	less than 1 gram fiber	230
Mission 96% Fat Free "Heart Healthy" Whole Wheat Flour Tortillas Plus! (1.5 oz) [1 Yellow Light Food and .5 Slimmer]	130	3	340
Mission Multi-grain Flour Tortillas Fajita Size (6 inch) [1 Yellow Light Food]	110	1	240
South Beach Diet Wraps Multi-grain or Whole Wheat (2 oz) [1 Yellow Light Food]	110	8	330
Thomas' Sahara Wraps 100% Whole Wheat (2 oz) [2 Slimmers]	170	4	310
WAFFLES			
Van's Original 97% Fat Free Waffles (1 waffle) [1 Slimmer]	72	2	160
Van's Original Berry Boost (1 Waffle) [1 Slimmer]	80	2	130
RICE			
White rice, steamed, ½ cup [1 Yellow Light Food]	103	0	1
ENGLISH MUFFINS			
Pepperidge Farm Whole Grain 100% Whole Wheat, (1 muffin) [1.5 Slimmers]	140	3	210

Food	Calories	Fiber (gm)	Sodium (mg)
ENGLISH MUFFINS *continued*			
Thomas' Hearty Grains 100% Whole Wheat (1 muffin) [1.5 Slimmers]	140	3	240
Trader Joe's British Muffins—Whole Wheat (1 muffin) [1.5 Slimmers]	140	5	230
BAGELS			
Pepperidge Farm Whole Grain 100% Whole Wheat Mini (1.5 oz) [1 Slimmer]	100	3	180
Sara Lee Heart Healthy Whole Wheat Cinnamon Raisin (½ bagel, 1.75 oz), [1.5 Slimmers]	125	3.5	170
Thomas' 100% Whole Wheat Mini-regular Oat Squares Bagel Bread (1 bagel, 2 oz) [1.5 Slimmers]	140	4	230
VitaMuffins (2 oz) (all flavors) [1 Slimmer]	100	4–5	130–140
VitaTops (all flavors) [1 Slimmer]	100	6	125–140
CRACKERS			
Kashi TLC Original 7 Grain Crackers (30 gm) [1.5 Slimmers]	130	2	160
Quaker Apple Cinnamon Rice Cakes (2 rice cakes, 30 gm) [1 Yellow Light Food]	100	0	0
Quaker Peanut Butter Chocolate Chip Rice Cakes (2 rice cakes, 30 gm) [1 Yellow Light Food]	120	0	140
Triscuits, Baked Whole Grain Wheat, Reduced Fat (29 gm) [1 Slimmer]	120	3	160
Wasa Crispbread, Hearty Whole Grain (28 gm) [1 Slimmer]	90	4	140

Food	Calories	Fiber (gm)	Fat (gm)	Sodium (mg)
POPCORN (less than 3 grams fat per serving)				
Healthy Choice Microwave Popcorn Butter or Natural Flavor (3 Tbsp, about 4 cups popped) [1 Yellow Light Food and .5 Slimmer]	130	5	2.5	290
Newman's Own Natural Mini Bags Microwave popcorn [1 Yellow Light Food]	100	4	2.5	210

Food	Serving Size	Calories	Sodium	Fiber
BEANS/BEAN MIXTURES				
Eden Green Lentils And Rice [1 Slimmer, Count as Carb or Protein Slimmer]	½ cup	120	120	2

Beans, Canned; see page 251-252 List B, Phase II (Beans Can Count as a Carb or Protein Slimmer)

Food	Calories	Fiber (gm)	Sodium (mg)	Sugar (gm)
CEREAL				
Barbara's Original Puffins [1 Slimmer]	90	5	190	5
Cheerios (28gm) [1 Yellow Light Food]	100	3	190	1
General Mills Fiber One Honey Clusters (1 cup) [2 Slimmers]	160	13	280	6
Grape Nuts (29 gm) [1 Yellow Light Food]	100	3.5	145	2
Kashi Nuggets (58 gm) [2 Slimmers]	210	7	260	3

Food	Calories	Fiber (gm)	Sodium (mg)	Sugar (gm)
CEREAL *continued*				
Kellogg's All-Bran with Extra Fiber (½ cup, 26 gm) [1 Slimmer]	50	13	120	0
Quaker Crunchy Corn Bran (¼ cup, 27 g) [1 Yellow Light Food]	90	5	240	6
Total (30 gm) [1 Yellow Light Food]	100	3	190	5
Wheaties (27 gm) [1 Yellow Light Food]	100	3	190	4
HOT CEREAL				
Kashi Instant Oatmeal, Raisin Spice (43 gm– 1 packet) [.5 Slimmer and 1 Yellow Light Food]	150	4	100	16
Nature's Path Instant Oatmeal, Apple Cinnamon (50 gm–1 packet) [2 Slimmers]	210	4	100	14
Nature's Path Instant Oatmeal, Regular (50 gm– 1 packet [2 Slimmers]	210	6	160	0
Quaker High Fiber Instant Oatmeal, Cinnamon Swirl [2 Slimmers]	160	10	210	7
Quaker High Fiber Instant Oatmeal, Maple and Brown Sugar [2 Slimmers]	160	10	260	7
Quaker Instant Oatmeal HIGH FIBER (2 servings Cinnamon Swirl) [2 Slimmers]	160	10	260	7

Food	Calories	Fiber (gm)	Sodium (mg)	Sugar (gm)
HOT CEREAL *continued*				
Quaker Instant Oatmeal Lower Sugar Apple and Cinnamon (31 gm) [1 Slimmer]	110	3	170	6
Quaker Instant Oatmeal, Cinnamon and Spice (46 gm–1 packet) [2 Slimmers]	170	3	250	15
Quaker Instant Oatmeal, Lower Sugar, Maple and Brown Sugar (34 gm–1 packet) [1 Yellow Light Food]	120	3	290	4
Quaker Instant Oatmeal, Weight Control, Banana Bread Flavor (45 gm–1 packet) [2 Slimmers]	160	4	260	1

List B (Phase II): Maintenance Plan Protein Slimmers
(Protein Slimmers from the Jumpstart Phase can also be chosen)

Food	Serving Size	Calories	Sodium	Fat	Fiber
CHEESE: FAT-FREE ≤240 mg Sodium per serving (Except cottage cheese <400 mg, ½ cup serving, limited to once a day)					
Borden, Fat Free [1 Yellow Light Food]	1 slice	30	320	0	0
Kraft, Fat Free Singles, average [1 Yellow Light Food]	1 slice	30	270–280	0	0
Kraft, Natural Fat Free Shredded Cheese, Cheddar [1 Yellow Light Food]	1 ounce	45	280	0	0
Polly-O Fat Free Mozzarella Cheese [1 Slimmer]	1 ounce	35	220	0	0

Food	Serving Size	Calories	Sodium ≤480 mg	Fat ≤1 gm
DELI POULTRY: (If you have more than 2 ounces of any deli meat, count the second two-ounce serving as a Yellow Light Food)				
Deli Poultry: (480–600 mg sodium) [1 Yellow Light Food]	2 ounces	50–80	480–600	1
Healthy Choice Oven Roasted Turkey Breast Deli Slices [1 Slimmer]	2 ounces	60	480	1
Jennie-O Sliced Turkey Breast, [1 Yellow Light Food]	2 ounces	50	590	1
Perdue Sliced Turkey Breast [1 Slimmer]	2 ounces	50	440	1

Food	Serving Size	Calories (Varies)	Sodium ≤240 mg; Always rinse canned fish
FISH/SHELLFISH: (If fish has more than 240 mg of sodium, count as 1 Yellow Light Food.)			
Alaska Snow Crab [1 Yellow Light Food]	2 ounces	63	382
American Tuna Albacore Canned in Water [1 Slimmer]	2 ounces	100	200
Bumble Bee or Chicken of The Sea Chunk or Solid Albacore Tuna Canned in Water [1 Slimmer]	2 ounces	75	231
Bumble Bee Prime Fillet Atlantic Pink Salmon [1 Slimmer]	2 ounces	80	171
Chicken of the Sea 50% Less Sodium Tuna, Light in Water [1 Slimmer]	2 ounces	60	125
Crown Prince Natural Solid Albacore White Tuna Canned in Water [1 Slimmer]	2 ounces	60	108

Food	Serving Size	Calories (Varies)	Sodium ≤240 mg; Always rinse canned fish
FISH/SHELLFISH *continued*			
Lobster, boiled or steamed, no butter [1 Slimmer]	2 ounces	56	216
Mussels, steamed, no added sauce or salt [1 Slimmer]	2 ounces	100	207
Phillips Jumbo Lump Canned Crab Meat [1 Protein Slimmer]	2 ounces	40	180
Starkist Albacore, Canned in Water or Pouch [1 Protein Slimmer]	2 ounces	73	191
Starkist Canned Tuna Creations, Herb & Garlic [1 Yellow Light Food]	2 ounces	80	320
Starkist Canned Tuna Creations, Sweet & Sour [1 Yellow Light Food]	2 ounces	80	270
Starkist Tuna Creations, Hickory Smoked in Pouch [1 Slimmer]	2 ounces	80	231
Starkist Tuna Creations Zesty Lemon Pepper, in Pouch [1 Slimmer]	2 ounces	60	217

Food	Serving Size	Calories	Sodium (mg)
BEANS AND LEGUMES			
Baked Beans (average all brands) [1 Yellow Light Food]	¼ cup	80	290
Beans, Refried (fat free and low-fat only) [1 Yellow Light Food]	½ cup *(Note: if ½ cup of beans has more than 600 mg sodium; stick to ⅓ cup serving)*	90–120	240–260

Food	Serving Size	Calories	Sodium (mg)
BEANS AND LEGUMES *continued*			
Bearitos Fat Free Refried Black Beans (Vegetarian) [1 Yellow Light Food]	½ cup *(Note smaller portion)*	70	530
Bearitos Fat Free Refried Green Chili Beans (Vegetarian) [1 Yellow Light Food]	½ cup	100	500
KFC Baked Beans (1 side order) [1 Yellow Light Food]	½ serving	100	350
Legumes, Lentils, and Split Peas (not green beans), canned [Count as either 1 Carb Slimmer or 1 Protein Slimmer]	½ cup	100	≤240 Rinse all beans to slash sodium by 40%

PREPARED MEATS AND FISH:
(See Convenience Prepared Foods, page 261–263)

TURKEY BURGERS: (See Convenience Prepared Foods page 261)

VEGGIE BURGERS: (See Convenience Prepared Foods page 261–263)

Food	Calories ≤100; 101–140 calories = 1.5 Slimmers	Saturated fat (g) ≤1 gram	Sugars (gm) ≤30 grams	Calcium (% DV)	Sodium (mg)
YOGURT (6 oz, unless noted)					
Horizon Organic Fat Free Fruit on the Bottom [1.5 Slimmers]	140	0	26	25	105
Lifeway Nonfat Kefir, Plain [1 Slimmer]	87	0	12	30	90
Oikos Organic Flavored Greek Yogurt (5.3 oz) [1.5 Slimmers]	120	0	14	17	60

Food	Calories ≤100; 101–140 calories = 1.5 Slimmers	Saturated fat (g) ≤1 gram	Sugars (gm) ≤30 grams	Calcium (% DV)	Sodium (mg)
YOGURT (6 oz, unless noted) *continued*					
Stonyfield Farm Organic Fat Free, all flavors (except Chocolate Underground) [1.5 Slimmers]	130	0	23	27	90–130
Stonyfield Farm Organic Low-Fat Flavored (except Caramel) [1.5 Slimmers]	130	1	22	26	105–110
Trader Joe's Nonfat Flavored [1.5 Slimmers]	130	0	23	25	97
Weight Watchers [1 Slimmer]	100	0	12	30	110
Yoplait Light & Thick and Creamy Light [1 Slimmer]	100	0	14	20	85–90

List C (Phase II): Maintenance Plan Mono Slimmers
(Count Each of the Following as 1 Mono Slimmer Unless Otherwise Noted)

Mono Slimmers	Serving Size	Calories ≤100 calories	Sodium ≤240 mg
Jif Creamy Peanut Butter	3 teaspoons	95	75
Jif Extra Crunchy Peanut Butter	3 teaspoons	95	65
Nut Butters	3 teaspoons	Varies	75–140
Nuts and Seeds, Salted (except peanuts)	6 teaspoons	100	60
Olives [0.5 Mono Slimmer]	7 small olives	30	210
Olives [0.5 Mono Slimmer]	3 large olives	30	175

Mono Slimmers *(continued)*	Serving Size	Calories ≤100 calories	Sodium ≤240 mg
Olives [1 Yellow Light Food]	6 large olives	60	350
Olives, chopped [1 Yellow Light Food]	4 tablespoons	40	300
PB2 (powdered peanut butter)	9 teaspoons	81	140
Peanuts, Salted	6 teaspoons	100	200
Peter Pan Creamy Peanut Butter	3 teaspoons	95	70
Skippy Creamy Peanut Butter	3 teaspoons	95	75
Smucker's Natural Peanut Butter Chunky	3 teaspoons	105	60
Tapenade [1 Yellow Light Food]	4 tablespoons	90	480
True North Almonds, Pistachios, Walnuts, Pecans, Lightly Roasted	4.5 teaspoons	100	83

List D: Maintenance Plan Convenience Prepared Foods
(Foods listed as Slimmers can count as a Carb or a Protein. Foods that are mainly protein are noted as Protein Slimmers and should not count as Carbs.)

Frozen Entrees	Serving Size	Calories ≤320	Fat ≤10 gm	Sat. Fat ≤2 gm	Sodium ≤400; 401–600 = 1 Yellow Light Food	Fiber ≥3 gm	Protein ≥5 gm
Amy's Bowls Brown Rice Black Eyed Peas and Veggies [2 Slimmers & 1 Yellow Light Food]	1 Bowl	290	11	1	580	8	11
Amy's Light in Sodium Brown Rice and Veggies Bowl [3 Slimmers]	1 Bowl	260	9	1	270	5	9

Frozen Entrees *(continued)*	Serving Size	Calories ≤320	Fat ≤10 gm	Sat. Fat ≤2 gm	Sodium ≤400; 401–600 = 1 Yellow Light Food	Fiber ≥3 gm	Protein ≥5 gm
Amy's Low in Sodium Vegetable Lasagna [2 Slimmers and 1 Yellow Light Food]	1 serving per container	290	8	3.5	340	4	15
Amy's Tofu Scramble with Hash Browns and Vegetables [2.5 Slimmers & 1 Yellow Light Food]	1 meal	320	19	3	580	4	19
Applegate Farms Natural Chicken And Apple Breakfast Sausage [0.5 Slimmer & 1 Yellow Light Food]	3 links (85 gm) Servings per con-tainer: About 3	140	8	2	450	0	15
Cedar Lane Garden Vegetable Enchiladas (Low Fat) [1.5 Slimmers]	1 enchi-lada (127 gm)	140	3	1.5	310	3	9
Cedar Lane Garden Vegetable Lasagna (Low Fat) [2 Slimmers]	5 oz (142 gm)	180	3	2	390	2	10
Healthy Choice Asiago Chicken Portobello [3 Slimmers]	1 meal (12.5 oz)	310	5	2	280	7	21
Healthy Choice Beef Merlot [1.5 Slimmers & 1 Yellow Light Food]	1 meal (284 gm)	220	6	1.5	580	5	17

Frozen Entrees (continued)	Serving Size	Calories ≤320	Fat ≤10 gm	Sat. Fat ≤2 gm	Sodium ≤400; 401–600 = 1 Yellow Light Food	Fiber ≥3 gm	Protein ≥5 gm
Healthy Choice Beef Pot Roast [2 Slimmers & 1 Yellow Light Food]	1 meal (11 oz)	310	7	3	500	5	15
Healthy Choice Blackened Chicken [2 Slimmers & 1 Yellow Light Food]	1 meal (11 oz)	310	6	1.5	600	6	16
Healthy Choice Classic Grilled Chicken BBQ [2 Protein Slimmers & 1 Yellow Light Food]	1 meal (11 oz)	270	3	1	430	7	15
Healthy Choice Country Herb Chicken [1.5 Slimmers & 1 Yellow Light Food]	1 meal (11.35 oz)	240	5	1.5	600	5	15
Healthy Choice Grilled Chicken Marinara [1.5 Protein Slimmers & 1 Yellow Light Food]	1 meal (284 gm)	250	4	1	550	5	20
Healthy Choice Grilled Monterey Chicken [2 Protein Slimmers & 1 Yellow Light Food]	1 meal (11 oz)	300	7	2.5	570	5	17

Frozen Entrees (continued)	Serving Size	Calories ≤320	Fat ≤10 gm	Sat. Fat ≤2 gm	Sodium ≤400; 401–600 = 1 Yellow Light Food	Fiber ≥3 gm	Protein ≥5 gm
Healthy Choice Honey Balsamic Chicken [2.5 Slimmers & 1 Yellow Light Food]	1 meal (12 oz)	350	6	1.5	460	4	13
Healthy Choice Lasagna Bake [1.5 Slimmers & 1 Yellow Light Food]	1 meal (9 oz)	240	4.5	1.5	600	5	11
Healthy Choice Lemon Pepper Fish [2 Protein Slimmers & 1 Yellow Light Food]	1 meal (10.7 oz)	310	4.5	1	440	5	13
Healthy Choice Macaroni and Cheese [1.5 Slimmers & 1 Yellow Light Food]	1 meal (9.1 oz)	210	4	2	600	4	9
Healthy Choice Roasted Chicken Marsala [1.5 Protein Slimmers & 1 Yellow Light Food]	1 meal (295 gm)	250	6	2	550	4	38
Healthy Choice Traditional Turkey Breast [2 Protein Slimmers & 1 Yellow Light Food]	1 meal (10.5 oz)	300	4	1	550	6	21
Kashi (Black Bean Mango) [2.5 Slimmers & 1 Yellow Light Food]	10 oz = 283 gm, Servings per container: 1	340	8	1	430	7	8

Frozen Entrees *(continued)*	Serving Size	Calories ≤320	Fat ≤10 gm	Sat. Fat ≤2 gm	Sodium ≤400; 401–600 = 1 Yellow Light Food	Fiber ≥3 gm	Protein ≥5 gm
Kashi Chicken Florentine [2 Slimmers & 1 Yellow Light Food]	1 entrée (283 gm)	290	9	4.5	550	5	22
Kashi Veggie Medley Pocket Bread Sandwich [2 Slimmers & 1 Yellow Light Food]	1 piece (156 gm) Servings per container: 1	280	7	1	570	6	1
Lean Cuisine Chicken Parmesan [2 Slimmers & 1 Yellow Light Food]	1 package	260	5	1.5	580	4	23
Lean Cuisine Deluxe Cheddar Potato [2 Slimmers & 1 Yellow Light Food]	1 package	260	7	3.5	600	4	14
Lean Cuisine Herb Roasted Chicken [1 Slimmer & 1 Yellow Light Food]	1 package (8 oz)	180	3.5	1	540	3	18
Lean Cuisine Roasted Chicken with Lemon Pepper Fettuccini [1.5 Slimmers & 1 Yellow Light Food]	1 package	230	6	2	580	2	16
Lean Cuisine Shrimp Alfredo [2 Slimmers & 1 Yellow Light Food]	1 package (9 oz)	260	5	2	590	3	18

Frozen Entrees *(continued)*	Serving Size	Calories ≤320	Fat ≤10 gm	Sat. Fat ≤2 gm	Sodium ≤400; 401–600 = 1 Yellow Light Food	Fiber ≥3 gm	Protein ≥5 gm
Schwan's Beef Stir Fry with Asian Noodles [1 Slimmer & 1 Yellow Light Food]	1 (Servings per container: 4)	190	4	1	520	4	14
Smart Ones Picante Chicken and Pasta [2 Slimmers & 1 Yellow Light Food]	255 gm	260	4	0.5	480	4	23
SmartOnes Broccoli and Cheddar Roasted Potatoes [1.5 Slimmers & 1 Yellow Light Food]	283 gm	220	6	3	480	5	9
SmartOnes Chicken Marsala with Broccoli [1 Slimmer & 1 Yellow Light Food]	255 gm	180	7	1	530	2	20
SmartOnes Honey Dijon Chicken [1.5 Slimmers & 1 Yellow Light Food]	241 gm	320	3.5	0.5	460	2	11
SmartOnes Penne Pollo [2 Slimmers & 1 Yellow Light Food]	283 gm	280	6	2.5	510	3	21

Frozen Entrees *(continued)*	Serving Size	Calories ≤320	Fat ≤10 gm	Sat. Fat ≤2 gm	Sodium ≤400; 401–600 = 1 Yellow Light Food	Fiber ≥3 gm	Protein ≥5 gm
SmartOnes Roasted Turkey Medallions w/ Mushroom Gravy [1.5 Protein Slimmers & 1 Yellow Light Food]	255 gm	220	1.5	0	550	3	13
SmartOnes Three Cheese Ziti Marinara [2 Slimmers & 1 Yellow Light Food]	255 gm	290	7	2.5	530	4	12
Trader Joe's BBQ Chicken Teriyaki [0.5 Protein Slimmer & 1 Yellow Light Food]	1 cup	150	3.5	1	570	0	18
Trader Joe's Chicken Tandoori with Spinach [3 Slimmers & 1 Yellow Light Food]	1 bowl (12 oz)	360	N/A	2	520	5	22
Trader Joe's Citrus Glazed Chicken [2 Slimmers & 1 Yellow Light Food]	1¾ cups	270	5	1	580	3	16
Trader Joe's Mandarin Orange Chicken [2.5 Slimmers]	1 cup	230	8	2	320	0	16
Trader Joe's Sweet and Sour Shrimp with Rice [2 Slimmers]	⅓ of package	190	0	0	350	2	8

Frozen Entrees (continued)	Serving Size	Calories ≤320	Fat ≤10 gm	Sat. Fat ≤2 gm	Sodium ≤400; 401–600 = 1 Yellow Light Food	Fiber ≥3 gm	Protein ≥5 gm
MISCELLANEOUS: To qualify, each should have less than 400 mg sodium and less than 2 grams saturated fat.							
Goya Fried Plantains [2 Slimmers]	3 med pieces (160 gm)	170	2	0.5	0	9	1
Morning Star Veggie Cakes Ginger and Teriyaki [1.5 Slimmers]	1 pattie (Servings per container: 4)	110	1.5	0.5	320	2	5
Trader Joe's Spanakopita Filled with Spinach, Ricotta, Feta [1 Slimmer]	1 piece (28 gm)	60	2	1	120	0	2
MEAT AND MEAT SUBSTITUTES							
Amy's Bistro Burger [1 Slimmer]	1 burger (71 gm)	90	2.5	0	340	2	5
Applegate Farms Organic Turkey Burger [1 Protein Slimmer & 1 Yellow Light Food]	1 burger (112 gm)	190	11	3	70	0	22
Applegate Farms Organic Chicken Strips [1 Protein Slimmer & 1 Yellow Light Food]	3 strips (84 gm) (Servings per container: About 2.5)	160	7	1.5	180	0	12

Frozen Entrees *(continued)*	Serving Size	Calories ≤320	Fat ≤10 gm	Sat. Fat ≤2 gm	Sodium ≤400; 401–600 = 1 Yellow Light Food	Fiber ≥3 gm	Protein ≥5 gm
MEAT AND MEAT SUBSTITUTES *continued*							
Bell and Evan's Breaded Chicken Breast Tenders [1 Protein Slimmer & 1 Yellow Light Food]	4 oz (113 gm) (Servings per container: About 3)	190	6	1	440	1	20
Bell and Evan's Fully Cooked Grilled Chicken Breast [1 Slimmer]	1 fillet 2.75 oz (78 gm)	80	0.5	0	260	0	18
Bell and Evan's Honey BBQ wings [1 Protein Slimmer & 1 Yellow Light Food]	3 pieces (132 gm) (Servings per con-tainer: 3)	160	8	2	240	0	17
Bell and Evan's Premium Chicken Burgers [1 Protein Slimmer & 1 Yellow Light Food]	4 oz (113 gm) (Servings per con-tainer: 4)	160	7	2	240	0	22
Boca Ground Crumbles [1 Slimmer]	57 grams (⅔ cup)	60	0.5	0	270	3	13
Gardenburger Black Bean Chipotle Veggie Burger [1 Slimmer]	1 burger	90	2.5	0	370	5	4

Frozen Entrees (continued)	Serving Size	Calories ≤320	Fat ≤10 gm	Sat. Fat ≤2 gm	Sodium ≤400; 401–600 = 1 Yellow Light Food	Fiber ≥3 gm	Protein ≥5 gm
MEAT AND MEAT SUBSTITUTES *continued*							
Morning Star Meal Starters Grillers Recipe Crumbles [1 Slimmer]	⅔ cup (Servings per container: About 6)	80	2.5	0	240	3	10
Morning Star Thai Burger [1 Slimmer]	1 burger (67 gm)	100	3.5	0.5	400	3	10
Oscar Mayer Canadian Bacon [1 Yellow Light Food]	2 oz	64	2	1	514	0	10
Perdue Shortcuts Carved Chicken Breasts [1 Yellow Light Food]	½ cup (71 gm) (2.5 oz)	90	2	0.5	500	0	17
Phillips Steamer Creations servings Steamed Spiced Shrimp [.5 Slimmer and Yellow Light Food]	4 oz (113 gm)	120	2	0	560	0	22

Convenience Bars: *(Bars with 121–150 calories count as 1.5 Slimmers and bars with 150–200 calories count as 2 Slimmers)*

Bars	Calories ≤200	Sat. Fat ≤1 (gm)	Fiber ≤3 (gm)	Sugar ≤12 gms, or NO Added Sugar	Sodium ≤130 (gm)	Protein (gm)
Clif Energy Bar (½ bar) [1 Yellow Light Food]	120 (limit to ½ bar)	0	2.5	11	50	5
CLIF ZBAR Kids Organic (All Flavors) [1 Slimmer], Bars containing 121–150 calories = 1.5 Slimmers]	120–150	1	3	9–12	75–125	3
KIND BAR Fruit and Nut Delight [1 Mono Slimmer & 1 Yellow Light Food]	170	1.5	3	12 (much naturally occurring from fruit)	25	6.5
KIND BAR Nut Delight [1 Mono Slimmer & 1 Yellow Light Food]	200	2	3	8	13	6.5
LARA BAR [2 Slimmers]	190	0.5	4	No added sugar	0	4–6

Soup: 1 cup	Serving Size	Sodium ≤400; 400–600 = 1 Yellow Light Food	Calories
Amy's Organic Soups—Light in Sodium (average of flavors) [1 Slimmer]	1 cup	290	100
Amy's Organic Butternut—Light in Sodium [1 Slimmer]	1 cup	290	100
Amy's Organic Minestrone Light in Sodium [1 Slimmer]	1 cup	290	90

Soup: 1 cup *(continued)*	Serving Size	Sodium ≤400; 400–600 = 1 Yellow Light Food	Calories
Amy's Organic Split Pea—Light in Sodium [1 Slimmer]	1 cup	280	100
Campbell's Select Healthy Request Chicken with Egg Noodles [1 Yellow Light Food]	1 cup	480	100
Campbell's Chunky Healthy Request Old Fashion Vegetable Beef [.5 Slimmer & 1 Yellow Light Food]	1 cup	480	110
Campbell's Select Healthy Request Savory Chicken and Long Grain Rice [.5 Slimmer & 1 Yellow Light Food]	1 cup	480	110
Campbell's Select Healthy Request and Campbell's Chunky Healthy Request (including microwave bowls) (average of flavors) [0.5 Slimmer & 1 Yellow Light Food]	1 cup	480	130
Health Valley Fat Free Corn and Vegetable [1 Slimmer]	1 cup	135	70
Health Valley Fat Free Italian Minestrone [1 Slimmer]	1 cup	210	91
Health Valley Fat Free Soups (average of flavors) [1 Slimmer]	1 cup	250	100
Health Valley Fat Free Tomato Vegetable [1 Slimmer]	1 cup	240	80
Health Valley No Salt Added Organic Black Bean [1.5 Slimmers]	1 cup	25	130
Health Valley No Salt Added Organic Lentil [1 Slimmer]	1 cup	25	100
Health Valley No Salt Added Organic Mushroom Barley [1 Slimmer]	1 cup	25	70
Health Valley No Salt Added Organic Potato Leek [1 Slimmer]	1 cup	35	70

Soup: 1 cup *(continued)*	Serving Size	Sodium ≤400; 400–600 = 1 Yellow Light Food	Calories
Health Valley No Salt Added Soups (average of flavors) [1 Slimmer]	1 cup	40	90
Health Valley Soups (average of flavors, NOT FAT FREE) [1.5 Slimmers]	1 cup	380	110
Healthy Choice Italian Style Wedding [.5 Slimmer & 1 Yellow Light Food]	1 cup	440	130
Progresso Healthy Favorites 50% Less Sodium [.5 Slimmer & 1 Yellow Light Food]	1 cup	460	110

The following soups are too low in calories to count as Slimmers. Since they are often used as flavoring agents like condiments, you'll count them as Condiments.

Campbell's Low Sodium Chicken Broth [1 Condiment]	1 can	140	24
Health Valley No Salt Added Fat Free Beef Flavored Broth [½ Condiment]	1 can	120	10
Healthy Valley No Salt Added Fat Free Chicken Broth [1 Condiment]	1 can	130	35

List E: Condiments

Try Bragg's Liquid Aminos as a soy sauce replacement! Use their 6-ounce Bragg's spray bottle and dilute with ⅓ distilled water; spray it on your food. 20 sprays = 1 Condiment

Condiments	Serving Size	Calories	Sodium (mg)
Annies Naturals Lite Honey Mustard Vinaigrette [½ Condiment]	1 tbsp	25	90
Big S Farms Smoke on the Mountain Habanero Salsa Medium [½ Condiment]	2 tbsp	10	50
Bouillon, Low Sodium [1 Condiment]	½ cube	5	25
Bragg Liquid Aminos [1 Condiment]	½ tsp	0	160
Campbell's Low Sodium Chicken Broth [1 Condiment]	1 cup	24	140

Condiments *(continued)*	Serving Size	Calories	Sodium (mg)
Chili Sauce [½ Condiment]	1.5 tbsp	9	94
Cindy's Kitchen Vidalia Onion And Cilantro [½ Condiment]	1 tbsp	30	70
Dijonnaise [½ Condiment]	1 tsp	5	70
Drew's All Natural Raspberry Dressing [½ Condiment or 3 Freebies]	1 tbsp	30	40
Garlic sauce [1 Condiment]	2 tsp	15 calories	185
Grated Parmesan [½ Condiment]	1 tbsp	22 calories	75
Health Valley No Salt Added Fat Free Beef Flavored Broth [½ Condiment]	1 cup	10	120
Healthy Valley No Salt Added Fat Free Chicken Broth [1 Condiment]	1 cup	35	130
Heinz No Salt Added Ketchup [½ Condiment or 2 Freebies]	1 tbsp	20	0
Honey [½ Condiment or 3 Freebies]	1½ tsp	30	0
Ken's Steakhouse Lite Sweet Vidalia Onion [½ Condiment or 3 Freebies]	2 tbsp	30	40
Ketchup [½ Condiment]	2 tsp	10	115
Kraft Reduced Fat Mayonnaise with Olive Oil [½ Condiment]	2 tsp	30	62
Litehouse Salsa Ranch Dressing [½ Condiment]	1 tbsp	25	100
Marie's Raspberry Vinaigrette [½ Condiment or 2 Freebies]	1 tbsp	20	30
Marie's Red Wine Vinaigrette [½ Condiment]	1 tbsp	30	100
Mayonnaise, Fat Free [½ Condiment]	1 tbsp	10	120
Mr. Spice Hot Wing! Sauce [½ Condiment or 2 Freebies]	1 tbsp	15	0

Condiments *(continued)*	Serving Size	Calories	Sodium (mg)
Mt. Olive Reduced Sodium Kosher Dill Strip [½ Condiment]	1 strip	5	120
Mustard [½ Condiment]	2 tsp	7	112
Nathan's Original Coney Island Deli Style Mustard [½ Condiment]	2 tsp	0	80
Naturally Fresh Apple Cranberry Walnut, Mixed Berry or Pomango [½ Condiment or 3 Freebies]	2 tbsp	30	5
Naturally Fresh Mandarin Ginger [½ Condiment]	2 tbsp	20	70
Naturally Fresh Raspberry Vinaigrette [½ Condiment]	1 tbsp	15	90
Old Cape Cod Fat Free Balsamic Vinaigrette [½ Condiment]	1 tbsp	15	85
Old Cape Cod Fat Free Honey Dijon [½ Condiment]	1 tbsp	25	65
Pickle Relish [½ Condiment]	1 tbsp	15	120
Salsa [½ Condiment]	1¼ tbsp	8	120
Salsa [1 Condiment]	2½ tbsp	8	240
Salsa, No Added Salt [½ Condiment]	4 tbsp	18	120
Sour Cream, Fat Free [½ Condiment or 2 Freebies]	2 tbsp	20	40
Soy Sauce (Less Sodium) [1 Condiment]	1 tsp	5	230
Sugar [½ Condiment or 3 Freebies]	2 tsp	30	0
Sugar-Free, Fat Free Hot Cocoa Carnation [1 Condiment]	1 packet	25	150
Trader Joe's Pineapple Salsa [½ Condiment]	2 tbsp	10	110

Condiments *(continued)*	Serving Size	Calories	Sodium (mg)
Westbrae No Salt Added Stoneground Mustard [Unlimited]	2 tsp	0	0
Whole Foods 365 Organic Raspberry Vinaigrette [½ Condiment or 3 Freebies]	1 tbsp	25	45
Wild Thymes Salad Refreshers [½ Condiment or 3 Freebies]	1 tbsp	30	5.5
Wishbone Salad Spritzers Caesar [½ Condiment]	10 sprays	15	85
Wishbone Salad Spritzers Italian or Asian Silk [½ Condiment]	10 sprays	10	100
Wishbone Salad Spritzers Red Wine Mist or Raspberry Bliss [½ Condiment]	10 sprays	10	95

Some of the Best Condiment Choices— Try These on Your Salads and Sandwiches

- **Balsamic vinegar.** Two teaspoons has 14 calories, 0 grams fat, and 2 milligrams sodium. (You don't even have to count it as a Freebie!)
- **Mustard.** One teaspoon has 10 calories, 0 grams fat, and 100 milligrams sodium.
- **Pickle relish.** One tablespoon has 21 calories, 0 grams fat, and 109 milligrams sodium.
- **Horseradish.** Two teaspoons has 4 calories, 0 grams fat, and 10 milligrams sodium.
- **Low-sodium light mayonnaise.** One-half tablespoon has 17 calories, 1.3 grams fat, and 27 milligrams sodium (the numbers may vary depending on brand).
- **Lemon.** Juice from ½ lemon has 8 calories, 0 grams fat, and 1 milligram sodium. (You don't even have to count it as a Freebie!)

Don't see your favorite condiment on the list? Check its Nutrition Facts label to see if it has less than 240 milligrams of sodium per serving. Remember, just as with salad dressings, you can make any condiment acceptable on the Maintenance Plan if you adjust the portion to meet the calorie (less than 60) and sodium (less than 240 milligrams) guidelines.

Appendix III:
Brand-Name Red Light Foods

(Notice some foods count as 2 Red Light Foods while others count as 2 Red Light Foods and a Yellow Light Food because they are so high in sodium.)

BLOATERS (These foods are salty or sugary and qualify as Bloaters; however, count them as Red Light Foods)	100-Calorie Serving (unless otherwise noted)	Sodium (mg) (If your food has more sodium than listed, don't eat it ... unless it's your birthday)	# of Red Light Servings
Baked Beans with Pork, canned, not rinsed, not drained	½ cup	601–700	2 Red Light Foods
Ham, deli, extra lean	2 oz	601–800	2 Red Light Foods
Hormel Canadian Bacon	2 oz	650	2 Red Light Foods
McDonald's Canadian Bacon (Limit to once a week) *(Note: Regular bacon is fattier and is a Flabber)*	2 oz	817	2 Red Light Foods & 1 Yellow Light Food
Oscar Mayer Deli Fresh Smoked Ham, 97% Fat-Free	2 oz	720	2 Red Light Foods
Oscar Mayer Sliced Oven Roasted Turkey Breast	2 oz	630	2 Red Light Foods
Oscar Mayer Sliced Smoked Turkey Breast	2 oz	630	2 Red Light Foods
Oscar Mayer Thin Sliced Deli Fresh Ham, Brown Sugar (Limit to once a week)	2 oz	830	2 Red Light Foods & 1 Yellow Light Food

BLOATERS (These foods are salty or sugary and qualify as Bloaters; however, count them as Red Light Foods)	100-Calorie Serving (unless other-wise noted)	Sodium (mg) (If your food has more sodium than listed, don't eat it … unless it's your birthday)	# of Red Light Servings
Poultry, Deli, lean	2 oz	601–800	2 Red Light Foods
Smoked, Cured, Aged and Salted Poultry Meats *(Note: For other fatty meats like salami, see Flabbers page X)*	2 oz	601–800	2 Red Light Foods
Soy products (veggie burgers, dogs or veggie "meats"); See Convenience Bloaters	varies	601–800	2 Red Light Foods

Bloater Cereals (>400 mg sodium per 120 calorie serving) Some foods qualify as Red Light Foods because they are Pluggers (not Bloaters) so they may contain ≤400mg of sodium/serving.	Calories (Eat a portion 120 calories or less)	≥400 mg sodium per 120-calorie serving	# of Red Light Servings
Crispix (29 gm)	110	210	1 Red Light Food
Special K (31 gm)	110	220	1 Red Light Food
Corn Flakes (28 gm)	100	200	1 Red Light Food
Rice Krispies (25 gm)	90	240	1 Red Light Food

Breads: Grains (Breads, Tortillas, Pitas, Prepared/Flavored Rice, Bagels, Couscous). Some foods qualify as Red Light Foods because they are Pluggers (not Bloaters) so they may contain ≤400mg of sodium/ serving. Please see 4 examples below.	Calories per serving (Limit to 120 calories or less)	>400	# of Red Light Servings
Bagel (2.5 oz [small])	½ bagel, (1.25 oz) 100 calories	379	½ bagel counts as 1 Red Light Food; 1 whole bagel is 2 Red Light Foods and 1 Yellow Light Food

Breads: Grains (Breads, Tortillas, Pitas, Prepared/Flavored Rice, Bagels, Couscous). Some foods qualify as Red Light Foods because they are Pluggers (not Bloaters) so they may contain ≤400mg of sodium/ serving.	**Calories per serving** (Limit to 120 calories or less)	**>400**	**# of Red Light Servings**
Croutons, seasoned	¾ cup, 92 calories	≥200 mg	1 Red Light Food
Mission Flour Tortillas (10-inch)	½ tortilla, 105 calories	315	1 Red Light Food
Pillsbury Oven Baked Dinner Rolls, Soft White, frozen	1 roll, 120 calories	170	1 Red Light Food
Sara Lee Hot Dog Bun, White Bread	1 bun, 120 calories	220	1 Red Light Food
White breads and rolls at restaurants	1 slice or roll, 100–120 calories	Varies (150–300)	1 Red Light Food

Convenience Food: SNACKS Some foods qualify as Red Light Foods because they are Pluggers (not Bloaters) so they may contain <600 mg of Sodium per serving	**Limit to 100-Calorie Portion** (See page 281 to account for calories over 100)	**600–800 mg =** **800–1,000 mg =**	**2 Red Light Foods Count as 2 Red Light Foods and 1 Yellow Light Food** (limit to once a week)
Movie Theatre Soft Pretzel	¼ large pretzel	500	1 Red Light Food
Salted Pretzels	1 oz	241–600 per serving	1 Red Light Food
Snyders of Hanover Mini Fat Free Pretzels	1 oz (20 pieces)	250	1 Red Light Food
Olives	18 small olives or 9 large	601	2 Red Light Foods
Rold Gold Classic Style Tiny Twists	1 oz	450	1 Red Light Food
Rold Gold Classic Style Rods	1 oz (3 rods)	610	2 Red Light Foods

Convenience Food: SOUPS Some foods qualify as Red Light Foods because they are Pluggers (not Bloaters) so they may contain <600 mg of Sodium per serving	Limit to 100-Calorie Portion (See page 281 to account for calories over 100)	600–800 mg = 800–1,000 mg =	2 Red Light Foods Count as 2 Red Light Foods and 1 Yellow Light Food (limit to once a week)
Campbell's Condensed Tomato Soup	½ cup	710	2 Red Light Foods
Campbell's Vegetable Beef Soup at Hand	1 container	930	2 Red Light Foods and 1 Yellow Light Food (Limit to once a week)
Canned Soups, non-cream based (creamed based are Flabbers)	¾ cup or ≤100 calories	600–800	2 Red Light Foods
Canned Soups, non-creamed based	¾ cup or ≤100 calories	≥800	2 Red Light Foods and 1 Yellow Light Food (limit to once a week)
Progresso Traditional Chicken Rice with Vegetables Soup	1 cup	870	2 Red Light Foods and 1 Yellow Light Food (limit to once a week)
Progresso Traditional Italian Style Wedding Soup	¾ cup	696	2 Red Light Foods

SUGARY BLOATERS: Sugary foods without added fat like jelly beans, Twizzlers, etc.	Each Serving = 100 Calories	Negligible Amounts of Sodium; Sugar Grams (gm) Are Listed Instead	# of Red Light Servings
CANDY			
Gummy Bears	11 gummy bears	14	1 Red Light Food
Jelly Beans, large size	10 pieces	20	1 Red Light Food
Jelly Belly Beans	25 pieces	16	1 Red Light Food
Jolly Rancher	4 pieces	15	1 Red Light Food
Skittles	½ serving size listed on bag	21	1 Red Light Food
Twizzlers, Strawberry, Chocolate, Cherry, or Licorice Twists	2¼ pieces	12	1 Red Light Food
Cookies, Cake, and Desserts (Even Fat Free)	1 oz (usually 1 small slice of cake or 2 small cookies)	varies	1 Red Light Food
Fat Free Fig Newtons	2 cookies	12	1 Red Light Food
Health Valley Fat Free Oatmeal Raisin Cookies	3 cookies	11	1 Red Light Food
Snackwell's Devil Food Cake Fat Free Cookies	2 cookies	14	1 Red Light Food
Jell-O (sugar added)	½ cup	30–60	1 Red Light Food
Yogurt (frozen)	½ cup (fat free)	60–150	1 Red Light Food
Cereals: Sugary, Refined Ones	¾ cup serving of Fruit Loops, Fruity Pebbles, Trix, Frosted Flakes, Corn Flakes, Cocoa Crispies, etc.	Varies (100–230)	1 Red Light Food

SUGARY BLOATERS: Sugary foods without added fat like jelly beans, Twizzlers, etc. *(continued)*	Each Serving = 100 Calories	Negligible Amounts of Sodium; Sugar Grams (gm) Are Listed Instead	# of Red Light Servings
DRINKS			
Gatorade	12 oz	24	1 Red Light Food
Soda, regular	8 oz	33	1 Red Light Food
ALCOHOL			
Wine	5 oz	see Alcohol (page 155)	1 Red Light Food
Beer	8 oz	see Alcohol (page 155)	1 Red Light Food
Light Beer	12 oz	see Alcohol (page 155)	1 Red Light Food
Liquor	1.5 oz	see Alcohol (page 155)	1 Red Light Food

NOTE: Count as 1 Red Light Food. Condiments with more than 600 mg of sodium per serving count as both of your Red Light foods for the day and are labeled.

Condiment	Serving Size	Calories	Sodium (mg)
Accent (Flavor Enhancer MSG)	½ tsp	0	320
Bacon Bits	1.5 tbsp	37	330
Barbeque Sauce (Kraft)	2 tbsp	40	420
Celery Salt	¼ tsp	0	448
Cocktail Sauce	2 tbsp	30	327
Creamy Cheese Sauce	2 fluid oz (4 tbsp)	45	510
Garlic Salt	¼ tsp	0	490

Condiment *(continued)*	Serving Size	Calories	Sodium (mg)
Gravy (canned)	¼ cup	33	333
Hollandaise Sauce	2 fluid oz (4 Tbsp)	140	260, 13 grams fat
Hot Sauce	2 tsp	0	250
Ketchup	2 tbsp	30	380
Ketchup (McDonald's)	3 packets	30	300
Meat Tenderizer	1 serving	0	400
Mustard	2 tbsp	20	340
Grey Poupon Classic Dijon Mustard	1 tbsp	15	360
Old El Paso Seasoning Taco Mix	2 tsp	15	560
Onion Salt	½ tsp	0	340
Pepperoncini Peppers	2 tsp	4	340
Salsa	4 Tbsp (2 fluid oz, ¼ cup)	20	400
Sliced Pickles	2 tsp	4	280
Steak Sauce	1 tbsp	15	280
Soy Sauce (Count as 2 Red Light Foods)	2 tsp	4	680
Soy Sauce, low sodium	1 tbsp	8	531
Sweet Pickle Relish	2 tbsp	50	280
Tabasco Sauce	2 tsp	0	250
Teriyaki Sauce (Count as 2 Red Light Foods)	1 tbsp	15	610
Tomato Sauce (average)	¼ cup		
Kraft Fat Free French Salad dressing	2 tbsp	45	290

Condiment *(continued)*	Serving Size	Calories	Sodium (mg)
Hidden Valley Fat Free Ranch Salad Dressing	2 tbsp	30	310
Kraft Fat Free Ranch Salad Dressing	2 tbsp	50	350
Walden Farms Sugar Free Italian Dressing	2 tbsp	20	400
Wendy's Honey Mustard Dressing	⅓ packet	95	116 sodium, 9 grams fat
Worcestershire sauce	5 Tbsp (⅓ cup)	40	260

100-Calorie Portions of Flabbers and Chubbers
(Each item qualifies as one of your two daily Red Light foods)

Most of the foods below are Flabbers. Some of the foods are Chubbers, however, regardless; they all qualify as one of your Red Light foods that should be limited to two each day.

Flabbers and/or Chubbers	Portion Size (100 Calories' Worth)
Biscuit, store/restaurant bought (Hardees, McDonald's Biscuits)	1 small
Candy Bar	⅓ bar or ½– ¾ oz
Chocolate Candy	¾ oz
Croissant	4½-inch x 4¾-inch; ½ croissant
Doughnut	3¼-inch diameter; ½ doughnut
French Fries	½ small order
Ice Cream	⅓ cup
Muffin	2½-inch diameter, 1½-inch high; 1 muffin

Flabbers and/or Chubbers *(continued)*	Portion Size (100 Calories' Worth)
Pie	9-inch diameter; 1/24 pie
Popcorn, Crunch 'n Munch	½ cup
Pop-Tart, Low-Fat (Kellogg's)	½ tart
Potato Chips	¾ oz, about 11 chips
Pudding	½ cup
Snack Bar (Balance Gold)	½ bar
Toaster Pastry	½ pastry
Yogurt, frozen	½ cup (fat-free is the best)
Butter, stick	1 flat tablespoon
Butter, pat	2½ pats
Whipped Cream	2 tbsp
COOKING FATS	
Bacon Fat	2 flat tsp
Beef Fat	2 flat tsp
Chicken Fat	2 flat tsp
Lard	2 flat tsp
Margarine (except trans free)	2 flat tsp
Coconut, shredded/grated	⅓ cup
SALAD DRESSINGS/SANDWICH SPREADS	
Blue Cheese, regular	1½ flat tbsp
Cream Cheese	2 flat tbsp
French, regular	1½ flat tbsp
Mayonnaise, regular	1 flat tbsp

Flabbers and/or Chubbers *(continued)*	Portion Size (100 Calories' Worth)
SALAD DRESSINGS/SANDWICH SPREADS *continued*	
Miracle Whip	2 flat tbsp
Ranch, regular	1½ flat tbsp
Tartar sauce, regular	1 flat tbsp
Thousand Island, regular	1½ flat tbsp
BEANS	
Baked, with added bacon or lard	¼ cup
Refried (not fat-free or low-fat)	¼ cup
CHEESE	
Brie	1 oz
Cottage, whole	⅓ cup
Goat Cheese (hard and semi-hard)	¾ oz
Gouda	1 oz
Mozzarella	1 oz
Parmesan, grated	4½ flat tablespoons or ¾ oz
Swiss	1 oz
Swiss, part skim, reduced fat	1 oz
Fish, canned in oil	1.5 oz
Deli Meats >3 grams fat	1 oz
Salami, Boar's Head Genoa	1 oz
Oscar Mayer Salami	1 oz

Convenience Foods, Frozen Entrées, and Prepared Meals

Convenience Foods: entrées, sandwiches, prepared meats, soups, main dishes, meals including frozen entrees	600–800 mg sodium ≤200 calories, especially bad if ≥ 2 grams saturated fat *or* <3 grams fiber	2 Red Light Foods
	600–800 mg sodium 220–300 calories (300 calories maximum)	2 Red Light Foods and 1 Yellow Light Food
	800–1,000 mg sodium 220–300 calories (300 calorics maximum)	2 Red Light Foods and 1 Yellow Light Foods (Limit to once a week.)

Red Light foods are limited to 300 calories; therefore, portion sizes of some foods in the list below have been adjusted to limit these damaging foods. Some foods are so troublesome that they are limited to once a week.

Convenience Red Light Food	Calories (No more than 300 calories)	Fat (>10 gm)	Fiber (<3 gm)	Protein (gm)	Sodium (mg)	# of Red Light Servings
Swanson's Meatloaf (Limit to once a week)	270	13	0	17	1,260	2 Red Light Foods and 1 Yellow Light (Limit to once a week)
Swanson's Carved Turkey (Limit to once a week)	250	11	0	10	1,100	2 Red Light Foods and 1 Yellow Light (Limit to once a week)
Boca Meatless Italian Sausage	130	6	1	13	650	2 Red Light Foods
Boca Meatless Italian Sausage	130	6	1	13	650	2 Red Light Foods
McDonald's Cheeseburger	300	12	2	15	750	2 Red Light Foods

Convenience Red Light Food	Calories (No more than 300 calories)	Fat (>10 gm)	Fiber (<3 gm)	Protein (gm)	Sodium (mg)	# of Red Light Servings
Soy products (ex: veggie burgers, dogs or veggie meats)	120–220	<10	varies	varies	600–800	2 Red Light Foods
Dixie's Diner Club, Meat (Not!) Chops, Deli Style	93	2.3	2.9	9.3	684	2 Red Light Foods
Swanson's Breaded Fish Fillet (¾ serving)	278	10.5	1.5	12	712	2 Red Light Foods and 1 Yellow Light Food
Swanson's Breaded Fish Fillet (¾ serving)	278	10.5	1.5	12	712	2 Red Light Foods and 1 Yellow Light Food

Appendix IV: Your Skinny Measurements: Track Your Progress

Date	Weight	Waistline (smallest area, in inches)	Butt/Hip (widest area, in inches)	Thigh (widest area, in inches)	Blood Pressure	Blood Cholesterol

Appendix V: The Food Log

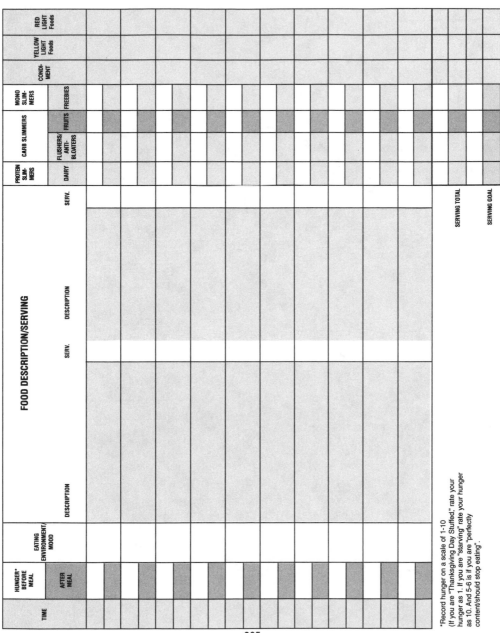

TIME	HUNGER* BEFORE MEAL / AFTER MEAL	EATING ENVIRONMENT/ MOOD	FOOD DESCRIPTION/SERVING DESCRIPTION	SERV.	DESCRIPTION	SERV.	PROTEIN SLIMMERS DAIRY	CARB SLIMMERS FLUSHERS/ ANTI-BLOATERS	FRUITS	MONO SLIMMERS FREEBIES	CONDI-MENT	YELLOW LIGHT Foods	RED LIGHT Foods
									SERVING TOTAL				
									SERVING GOAL				

*Record hunger on a scale of 1-10
(If you are "Thanksgiving Day Stuffed," rate your hunger as 1. If you are "starving" rate your hunger as 10. And 5-6 is if you are "perfectly content/should stop eating".

285

References

Hills, S. "New Sea Salt with a Larger Punch." Food Navigator.com. Accessed 6/20/08.

Merriam–Webster's Online Dictionary. http://www.merriam–webster.com/dictionary/salt. Accessed 6/26/08.

Salt Works. "History of Salt." http://www.saltworks.us/salt_info/si_HistoryOfSalt.asp. Accessed 6/10/2008.

Stephens, A. "Well Seasoned: How salt can actually be good for you." http://www.independent.co.uk/lifestyle/health=and=familes/health=news/well=seasoned=how=salt=can=actually=be=good=for=you=771.775.html. Accessed 7/8/2009. January 2008.

Index

About the Authors

Tammy Lakatos Shames and **Elysse ("Lyssie") Lakatos,** also known as The Nutrition Twins®, are registered dietitians and personal trainers who share more than identical features; they share a mission to help people improve their health through lifestyle-focused behavior modification. What began as a passion for improving the way people feel inside and out morphed into the founding of an innovative nutrition company, The Nutrition Twins®.

Tammy and Lyssie have become known for their unique approach to nutritional counseling, corporate lecturing, writing, making media appearances, and consulting multi-national food companies. The Lakatos sisters have worked with hundreds of corporations and serve as the exclusive nutritionists for NBC's celebrities and employees at Rockefeller Plaza in New York City.

Lyssie and Tammy are coauthors of their first book, *Fire Up Your Metabolism: 9 Proven Principles for Burning Fat and Losing Weight Forever* (Simon and Schuster).

The Twins have been featured regularly as the nutrition experts on *Good Morning America,* the Discovery Health channel, Fox News Channel, NBC, Bravo, WABC-TV, WPIX-TV, CBS, The Learning Channel, FitTV, Oxygen Network, and Fox & Friends. Tammy and Lyssie have become sought-after contributors by many print and online publications. They have been featured on the cover of *Woman's World* magazine and have appeared in magazines such as *Cosmopolitan, Self, Good Housekeeping, Vogue, InStyle, Glamour, People,* and *O Magazine.* In addition, the sisters serve as the exclusive nutritionists for FitTV online.

Tammy and Lyssie reside in New York City where they assist celebrities, professional athletes, and everyday people in attaining their personal health-related goals. Former soccer and speedskating competitors, the twins now enjoy running and pumping iron and Tammy chases after her twin toddler girls to keep fit.